Be a Survivor™
Your Guide to Breast Cancer Treatment

Be a Survivor™
Your Guide to Breast Cancer Treatment

Vladimir Lange, M.D.

ISBN 0-9663610-0-8

Library of Congress Card #98-84908

Printed in the United States of America

Be a Survivor™
Your Guide to Breast Cancer Treatment

VLADIMIR LANGE, M.D.

Presented by:

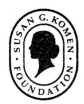

The Arkansas Chapter of the
Susan G. Komen Breast Cancer
Foundation

Phone 1-800-I M AWARE

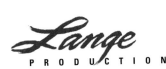

Lange PRODUCTIONS

LOS ANGELES

To Mandy,
Chad, and Christy

Table of Contents

Consultants on *Be A Survivor*™ Programs

Terri Ades
Leslie Botnick, M.D.
R. James Brenner, M.D., J.D.
Aman Buzdar, M.D.
Cathy Coleman, R.N., O.C.N.
James D. Cox, M.D.
Helen Crothers, M.S.W.
Bradford W. Edgerton, M.D.
Carol Fabian, M.D.
Barbara Fowble, M.D.
William H. Goodson, III, M.D.
William H. Hindle, M.D.
Soram Singh Khalsa, M.D.
Lydia Komarnicky, M.D.
Jean Lynn, R.N.B.S., O.C.N.
Silvana Martino, D.O.
Stephen Mathes, M.D.
Beatrice Mautner, R.N.
Shirley McKenzie, R.N., P.H.N.
Candace Moorman, M.P.H.
Betsy Mullen
Karen Schmitt, R.N.
Stuart J. Schnitt, M.D.
Barbara L. Smith, M.D., Ph.D.
David Spiegel, M.D.
Lisa Summerlot, R.N., O.C.N.
Victor Vogel, M.D.
Deane Wolcott, M.D.

Acknowledgments

This book is based on more than a decade of professional experience creating educational programs about breast cancer, and on my personal experience dealing with breast cancer as the husband of a survivor.

A list of the names of all those who helped me, encouraged me, and taught me during these years would be longer than the book itself. I thank all of them for their time and kind support.

Several of them deserve special gratitude.

My most sincere thanks go to my valued consultants, recognized experts in their fields, who contributed their time and knowledge to make this book informative, accurate, and up-to-date. It is particularly gratifying that two of them, William Goodson and David Spiegel, are my friends and classmates from Harvard Medical School days. Bill reviewed the manuscript from cover to cover, with surgical precision, spotting areas that needed enhancement.

Three of the consultants, Lisa Summerlot, Karen Schmitt, and Candace Moorman, contributed their extensive experience in dealing with breast cancer patients. They helped me not only with the facts, but also with my writing style.

Lisa helped write the scripts and overcome the production stumbling blocks for many of the video programs on which the CD-ROM and the book are based.

Karen reviewed the entire CD-ROM from introduction to credits, mercilessly pointing out where my style did not measure up.

And Candace challenged me by saying that the world did not need another breast cancer book, then rewarded me by admitting that she wished she had this book when she was diagnosed with breast cancer herself.

Thank you! Each of you made the book better.

I also want to thank the survivors and their partners who gave freely of their time and candidly shared their stories. Two survivors deserve extra special thanks.

Betsy Mullen, diagnosed at age 33, contributed her experience, not only as a survivor, but also as the founder and president of WIN, the Women's Information Network Against Breast Cancer.

Cathy Masamitsu, diagnosed at age 32, helped bring the *Be A Survivor* program to the attention of her viewers on the *Home & Family Show*, where she is a producer and reporter.

Thanks are also due to Deane Wolcott, M.D. and Valen Watson for helping generate interest in the right circles when the CD-ROM was being developed, and to Linda Gordon for encouraging the "book idea" even before it was an idea.

Thanks to my efficient and talented team for working so diligently during production of all the programs on which this book is based. In the final phase, Rob Elhardt oversaw the metamorphosis of the 12-hour CD-ROM into the book you are now reading.

Special thanks to Jim Robie of Los Angeles for generously contributing his talent in creating the design and layout for the book.

My love and gratitude to our children, Chad and Christy, for always being there for me, for their Mom, and for each other. And most of all, my love and admiration to my wife Mandy, who has survived her battle and remains a shining beacon, a powerful inspiration, and a valued critic.

Introduction

The diagnosis of breast cancer is a shattering experience. I know. My wife was diagnosed with the disease ten years ago. We thought our world would come to an end. My wife struggled with the possibility of losing her life. I was faced with losing the woman I love, and confronted by the prospect of raising two teenagers alone.

Both of us are physicians. She is a pediatrician, and I was an emergency room doctor. We were well-read (at least in medical matters), cool and composed under stress, rational adults able to handle crises — or so we thought. Despite excellent care from breast cancer experts who were also our colleagues and friends, we were totally overwhelmed — by the diagnosis and by the torrent of information that was thrown at us. We had learned about radiation therapy, chemotherapy, and surgery in medical school. Yet we sat there wondering if these people were speaking Greek — or perhaps Latin. It was weeks before we were able to unravel all the details and ramifications, and begin deciding on a course of treatment.

This book, and the video and CD-ROM on which it is based, were created to help you and your loved ones better understand what you are facing, and participate in your treatment and recovery.

The book is a balanced, objective presentation of the latest information, developed in consultation with dozens of top experts in the field, that will help you understand the facts about breast cancer. To this we added candid comments by patients and their partners — the women and men who have "been there," and whose voices can help you understand your own feelings and frustrations at this difficult time.

Facts to Remember About Breast Cancer

- Breast cancer is not a death sentence — 98% of those diagnosed are successfully treated if the cancer is detected early.
- Breast cancer can often be treated with breast-conserving surgery — preserving the natural appearance of the breast.
- Excellent options for reconstruction are available if mastectomy is necessary.
- In most cases there is no need to rush your decisions. Take time to learn as much as you can, and to decide what choices are best for you.
- A positive attitude and active participation will improve the outcome of your treatment. Be resolved that you will survive this challenge.

How To Use This Book

The book can be used in conjunction with the *Be A Survivor* ™ CD-ROM or video, where you can actually hear the patient interviews, and see the animated graphics and film clips of the procedures. However, even if you don't have the CD-ROM or the video, the book alone is still an excellent source of information.

Each chapter includes lists of questions you might want to ask your healthcare professionals. For your convenience, these questions are repeated at the end of the book. You can take them, or the whole book, with you on office visits to help you communicate more effectively.

We've tried to lay out the book in a way that mirrors your path through treatment and recovery.

First, we've provided a few suggestions on how to cope with your diagnosis — coming to grips with your feelings so you can think and evaluate the facts. There are tips on how to tell your family, friends, and co-workers about your diagnosis, and how to assemble a network of support to help you get through the tough times.

Next is an overview of breast cancer treatment. If you only read one section in this book, make sure it's this one. It will help you understand how the different aspects of your treatment fit together, and help you evaluate your options.

The majority of the book consists of a detailed description of the various procedures and treatments you may encounter: diagnostic procedures, such as biopsy; surgery, including mastectomy, lumpectomy, and reconstruction techniques; and adjuvant therapies, such as radiation, hormonal therapy, and chemotherapy. We have included information on complementary treatments, such as relaxation, visualization, and acupuncture, which may be valuable additions to your battle with cancer.

The book also will help you make a smooth transition from treatment to recovery, both emotionally and physically. It will show you how to follow-up with your doctor, and how to keep yourself healthy.

The last chapter of the book is devoted to your partner — husband, boyfriend or special man or woman in your life. It not only teaches how to provide support for you, but also speaks directly to the needs of your partner during this time.

At the end of the book we've included several useful reference sections, such as a glossary of important breast cancer terms, a library listing of other books and videos on the subject, and a resource section with names, numbers, and website addresses of organizations and programs that can help you.

We wish you a speedy recovery.

CHAPTER 1

Facing Breast Cancer

"You have breast cancer."

These are perhaps the most frightening words you've ever heard. But it is important for you to realize that a diagnosis of breast cancer is not a death sentence. Breast cancer is a very treatable disease, and survival rates today are higher than ever before. There are more than one and a half million women who have been handed the same diagnosis years ago, and are still leading happy, productive lives. So try to resolve, right now, that you will do everything you can to be successful in your battle against breast cancer.

On the following pages we will discuss the initial steps you need to take:

- Understand your feelings
- Decide how, when, and with whom to share the news
- Assemble a support network
- Gather the information you need
- Actively participate in planning your treatment

UNDERSTANDING YOUR FEELINGS

The first thing to do is take time to get in touch with your feelings. Cry, get angry, shout. Show whatever emotion helps you, because there is no right or wrong response, and different women react in different ways.

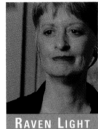

RAVEN LIGHT

When the doctor said, "Yes, it's malignant," my mind went kind of blank. "What am I going to do; How am I going to pay the rent? This can't be happening to me. Who's this happening to?" And then I felt myself kind of disassociate, and I became very coldly rational.

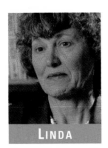

LINDA

Terry was away. He was on a film shoot. And so, I asked a girlfriend to be there when I got home. He called and I had to tell him over the phone. He came home the next day. It was hard.

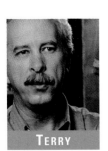

TERRY

Everything was tossed upside down. I wanted to rush back to her. I was pretty broken up. I didn't really know what it meant to have breast cancer. It could be something that we could get through or it could be a major crisis to her health.

The first few weeks after your diagnosis may be the hardest to handle. No matter how strong you are, you may find that you have trouble managing the emotional roller coaster.

Find someone you can talk to about your emotions. This should be a mature, well-adjusted person who can listen without passing judgment. Sometimes very close friends or family members may be too involved in the situation to remain objective. At least initially, it may be best to speak to someone who is not dealing with their own emotions or who has a need to "make it all better."

A good resource for talking about your feelings, as well as practical concerns, may be another woman who had breast cancer, or an organized group of breast cancer survivors who meet regularly to offer mutual support and a forum for open communication.

Don't be embarrassed to seek professional help. Group or individual counseling can help you come to grips with your feelings, so you can start on the road to recovery.

SHARING THE NEWS

Telling Your Partner

Your partner probably will be affected by your diagnosis as much as you. In some ways your partner's role will be particularly difficult because it will involve managing new emotions, as well as shouldering the task of being your key supporter.

Couples may have difficulty adjusting to the role changes that are sometimes necessary. A partner who was responsible for only part of the daily activities may now become the sole breadwinner and homemaker, preparing dinner, changing the bedding and dressings, and providing companionship and emotional support. The sheer weight of these responsibilities can disrupt normal relationships, use up the time needed for rest and recreation, and deprive everyone of opportunities to express anxiety and resentment.

A partner's concern or fears also can affect your sexual relationship. Some may worry that physical intimacy will harm the person who has cancer.

Others may fear that they might "catch" the cancer or be affected by the drugs. Many of these issues can be cleared up by talking about misunderstandings. Both you and your partner should feel free to discuss sexual concerns with your doctor, nurse, or other counselor who can give you the information and the reassurance you need.

Most couples find ways to face and overcome the stress cancer places on their relationship. It is very important that you involve your partner as soon as possible, so the two of you can share your feelings and your fears, and establish lines of communication for the weeks and months to come. This will help you find strength in each other, and work together to establish a new and comfortable routine.

Telling Your Family

The people who are close to you also will be affected by your news. They too may need to be angry, cry, and express their emotions. It's a natural part of adjusting to your diagnosis. It will help both you and them to talk openly about each other's feelings. Open communication from the start will go a long way toward strengthening the bonds with your loved ones, and securing the support you'll need.

Telling the Children

You will probably want to shield your children from pain, but don't underestimate their ability to pick up signals that all is not well. Children's insight is greater than most people realize, and trying to keep a complex situation such as cancer a secret, is practically impossible. A simple and straight-forward explanation, geared to each child's age and ability to understand, will keep them from imagining situations worse than the reality. This is especially important for younger children, who may feel responsible, in some way, for your illness.

Some adults still remember the feelings of rejection they suffered when they were not included in the family's handling of a situation. Here is a school essay written by a twelve-year old daughter of a woman undergoing breast cancer treatment. Her parents attempted to protect her from what they considered unnecessary pain by minimizing the severity of the condition. She protected them from her own feelings by not sharing the essay with them until years later.

QUESTIONS TO ASK YOUR DOCTOR:

☐ What should I tell my loved ones about my condition?

☐ May I bring members of my family, or a friend, to talk to you directly?

☐ Can you refer me to a counselor or to a support group specializing in breast cancer issues?

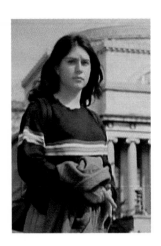

My father's face is red and bloated. A plate of blackened hamburgers is trembling in his hands. If he clutches the sides of the dish any tighter, it will collapse into splinters on the tablecloth in front of him. I am looking up at his thick, wrinkled forehead as his mouth opens and closes, spilling angry words: How could I be so careless? Didn't I realize they were burning? I do not offer any explanation about my carelessness. I just look down at my sneakers and moan.

There is a deafening crash as my father slams the plate of burned food onto our dining room table. The table shakes and the silverware rattles. My father, my mother, my teenage brother and I slide noiselessly into our chairs as if we are performing a solemn ritual. When I glance up at my father's swollen, contorted face, I can feel hot anger burning at the top of my stomach and shooting up into my throat. There is a familiar, irritating pain in my forehead and around my eyes. I strain to hold back the tears that I know are waiting, but the liquid collects in my eyelashes, forming droplets that slowly pull themselves down my cheeks.

"Why are you crying?" My father's voice is louder than he expects it to be. The look on his face tells me that he knows I am not crying over burned hamburgers. He knows exactly why I am crying. He would cry those same frustrated tears if his ego would let him.

I am crying because my mother has cancer. It is the third month of her chemotherapy; the third month we have had to pretend that our family is still as strong as it ever was, that my mother's illness is just a temporary setback. But tonight the perfect composure of my family is breaking down underneath the weight of my mother's disease. Our family is too tired to pretend anymore.

I am tired of not being able to be a normal twelve year old. I am tired of telling my mother that everything is fine, that she doesn't have to be at my soccer game, that it is OK if she is too sick to eat a piece of my birthday cake. It is no longer fine. Our family cannot survive without my mother. It does not matter that my brother had learned to do laundry while my father goes to PTA meetings and I teach myself how to cook. We can no longer smile while we take on new roles in the household that we know could be permanent. We cannot bear to think that my mother may die, but we cannot hide the fact that we are thinking it.

"Why are you crying?" My father's words are still reverberating in my brain as I search for a safe place to stare so I do not have to face the sadness

in the room.   I hear a tiny sound, a low whimper escaping from my mother's side of the table.   I glance over at her and watch her hunched shoulders moving rhythmically up and down as she fidgets with the tablecloth.   She lifts her pale face and looks around the dining room as if she too is wondering where the sound is coming from.   Her eyelids are dark red and tears are slipping effortlessly down her face.

It is the first time I have seen my mother cry — not just since her diagnosis, but since I can remember.   I want to look away, but I keep staring, waiting for my body to confirm that the events taking place are real.   My mother shakes her head slowly, as if she is scolding herself for revealing the pain she has been harboring underneath her confident exterior.

"Oh God, I'm so sorry."   The words come tumbling from my mouth.   "I'm so sorry, I'm so sorry."   I keep vomiting the words.   I run to my mother's side, frantic, hoping I can get to her fast enough to return her to the moment before she began suffering.   "I'm sorry, Mommy.   I'm sorry."   I hug her tighter than I ever have before, letting her hair stick to my wet cheek.   "I'm so sorry."   The words are not even mine anymore.   They are escaping from a place in my body that I never knew existed.   I am not thinking about anything else, about what my father and brother must be thinking, about what it will be like after this moment.   "I'm sorry..."

I'm sorry that I've been selfish, sorry that I got mad when you weren't excited about my report card, sorry I refused to go with you to your first dose of chemotherapy, sorry that I laughed at your new wig, sorry that I ran away when you threw up in the kitchen sink.   I'm sorry I didn't know how you were suffering.

I am holding my mother's trembling body.   I rest my chin in the crevasse of her shoulder the way I used to when she knelt down to hug me. The room and its contents no longer exist. My mother and I are alone, clinging to each other, and I am wishing that I could heal her.   I press my lips to her ear and whisper, "Mommy, please don't die."

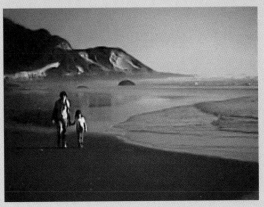

Dealing with Problems in the Family

Cancer is a blow to every family it touches. How you handle it is determined to a great extent by how you have functioned as a family in the past. Families who are used to sharing their feelings with each other usually are able to talk about the disease and the changes it brings. Families in which each member solves problems alone or in which a single person has played the major role in making decisions, might have more difficulty coping.

Children, especially, may have difficulty coping with cancer in a parent. Some fear the loss of the parent or begin to imagine their own death. In addition to this upheaval, children often are asked to "play quietly," to perform extra tasks, or to be understanding of others' moods beyond the maturity of their years.

Younger children may resent lost attention. Teenagers can feel torn between expressing independence and a need to remain close to the sick parent. Discipline problems can arise. Parents may not have the emotional energy to provide the usual support, love, and authority.

It may help if a favorite relative or family friend can devote extra time and attention to the children to help maintain normal family routines as much as possible. Events like trips to the zoo are important, but so is helping with homework, or attending the basketball awards banquet.

In more difficult situations, individual or family counseling can help with the stress. Your physician, a hospital social worker, or hospital psychologist are good sources for referrals to psychologists, psychiatrists, or other mental health professionals trained to counsel individuals and families affected by cancer.

Dealing with Friends

Friends can be an excellent source of help and support, particularly if you keep them informed, and help them help you. Some friends will deal well with your illness and will provide gratifying support. Some will be unable to cope with the possibility of your death, and will disappear from your life. Most will want to help, but may be unsure of how to go about it, and will be waiting for clues from you about where to begin.

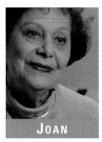

JOAN

When you get that diagnosis, go ahead and cry your eyes out. Cry your eyes out right then, so that you're not bottling up that emotion. It's so terrifying, that for a while you feel as though you're in a fog, and that if you come out of this fog, something terrible is going to happen. So, cry it, vent it, talk it out, and then find out what you can do to help yourself.

You may be the one who will have to take the initiative in reestablishing contact. Telephone those who don't call you. Ask for simple things — to run an errand, prepare a meal, come and visit. These small acts bring friends back into contact and help them feel useful and needed.

Beyond the immediate circle of people who are close to you, or who have something positive to offer, telling others about your diagnosis should be on a "need to know" basis. No one is entitled to have information you don't want to give out. Women have gone through full breast cancer treatments, including surgery, while their co-workers remained unaware of what was going on.

Dealing with Employers

When you return to work, you may encounter discrimination on the grounds that people who have cancer take too many sick days, are poor insurance risks, or will make co-workers uncomfortable.

How can you deal with these issues? Under Federal law, most employers cannot discriminate against handicapped workers, including people with cancer. These laws apply to Federal employers, employers that receive Federal funds, and private companies with 25 or more employees. State laws also forbid discrimination based on handicap, but only some protect people with cancer.

If you are applying for a job with a government agency or a firm with government contracts, and believe you did not get the job because of your cancer, you can file a complaint with the Department of Justice.

If you believe you were discriminated against by a private employer because of your cancer, you should file your complaint with the closest regional office of the Equal Employment Opportunities Commission.

GOVERNMENT JOBS

You are protected under Section 504 of the Federal Rehabilitation Act of 1973, and by the Americans with Disabilities Act of 1990. Write directly to the agency involved, or contact the Civil Rights Division of the U.S. Department of Justice, Washington, DC. (202) 724-2235.

PRIVATE SECTOR

To obtain the location of your regional Equal Employment Opportunities Commission office and find out exactly what to do, call (800) USA-EEOC.

Find out more about your rights:

- Your local American Cancer Society offices have state-specific information about cancer and employment discrimination.
- Your social worker may know about laws in your state and also can tell you which state agency is in charge of protecting employee rights.

- Your state's Department of Labor Office of Civil Rights.
- The National Coalition for Cancer Survivorship offers information and limited attorney referrals.
- Regional or national offices of the Civil Liberties Union.
- Your representative's or senator's office has information about Federal and State laws. If you are not sure who represents your district, call your local library or local chapter of the League of Women Voters.
- The local branch of the American Bar Association.

ASSEMBLING YOUR SUPPORT NETWORK

One of your first steps should be to establish a network of people who can help you. This network can include your loved ones, peer support groups, and your healthcare professionals.

Friends and Family

Your loved ones will provide the emotional support and closeness you need, and help you sort out facts and fears.

Try to select one person — your husband, partner, or best friend — who will accompany you when you meet with your doctors or go to your treatments. This companion can help you ask questions, remember information, or write down instructions.

He or she also can become the center of your support network, acting as your sounding board, helping you evaluate information and make decisions, coordinating support from friends and family, and at times shielding you from excessive attention.

Support Groups

One of the most beneficial things you can do is join a support group. Support groups are groups of people who meet regularly, under the guidance of a trained facilitator, to discuss the participants' concerns.

Programs are organized in a variety of ways. Some groups meet only a few times; others are long-term, enabling members to work through problems. Some are composed of people with the same disease site (breast or colon

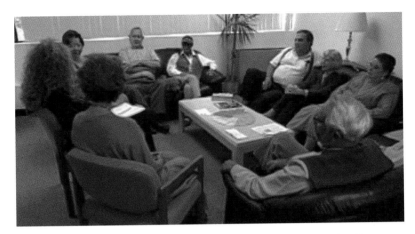

cancer patients), others by patient age or background. Some are just for patients; others include family or other special people.

Support groups give you a chance to openly discuss your thoughts with others who are going through the same experience. Many hospitals consider some form of group counseling to be part of the standard treatment — as necessary as an exercise class, for example.

In 1989, a landmark study by Dr. David Spiegel at Stanford University proved the benefits of psychosocial therapy for patients with metastatic breast cancer. Eighty six women were divided into two groups. Half were given standard medical care (radiation or chemotherapy) while the other half received the same care and also met once a week in a group therapy session.

The women in the support group not only reported less anxiety, depression, and pain than the group who received only standard medical care, but also lived almost twice as long!

Your Healthcare Team

Cancer is a complicated disease and no single physician can be an expert in all aspects of the treatment. Developing a treatment plan is a complex task that will involve a number of healthcare professionals — a real team of experts — who will give you their recommendations regarding surgery, chemotherapy, and radiation.

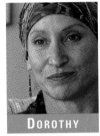

DOROTHY

My group really offers me an opportunity to share my truest feelings, my most private feelings, and my greatest fears in a place where there's support, caring, friendship, and the courage of other people leading you forward.

15

Some hospitals and cancer centers already have teams of breast cancer experts, called multidisciplinary teams. If yours doesn't, the National Cancer Institute, the American Cancer Society, the Susan G. Komen Foundation, or the Y-ME organization have resources that will help you find healthcare professionals to add to your team, or to give you a second opinion.

You may want to seek out specialists in specific areas of interest to you, such as chemotherapy or breast reconstruction. Or you may establish a relationship with a generalist who will help you sift through the information you are receiving, or whom you could call with questions that crop up at a time when your regular team is not available.

Here, in alphabetical order, is a list of the specialists who may be involved in your treatment.

Anesthesiologist: Administers drugs or gasses which put you to sleep before surgery.

Clinical Nurse Specialist: A nurse with training or knowledge in a specific area, such as post-operative care, chemotherapy, or radiation therapy.

Medical Oncologist: A doctor who administers anti-cancer drugs or chemotherapy.

Pathologist: A doctor who examines the tissue removed during a biopsy, and issues a report to help you and your doctor choose the most effective treatment.

Personal Physician: The doctor who will be responsible for coordinating your treatment. Your personal physician may be a surgeon, radiation oncologist, medical oncologist, or family physician.

Physical Therapist: A specialist who helps with post-surgical rehabilitation using exercise, heat, or massage.

Plastic Surgeon: A doctor specializing in cosmetic surgery, such as breast reconstruction after mastectomy.

QUESTIONS TO ASK YOUR DOCTOR:

☐ Could you give me the names of specialists you think I should see?

☐ How about another set of names so I can choose the specialist(s) I like best?

☐ Is there a multidisciplinary breast cancer team in the facility where you practice?

☐ Tell me about your, or your colleagues' experience in dealing with breast cancer.

Radiation Therapy Technologist: A specially-trained technologist who works under the direction of the Radiation Oncologist to administer external radiation treatment.

Radiation Oncologist: A physician specifically trained in the use of high energy x-rays to treat cancer.

Social Worker: A trained professional who can deal with social and economic aspects of treatment, such as helping find a support group or solving an insurance issue.

Surgeon: A doctor specializing in surgery, who will do the operation to remove the cancer.

Getting a Second Opinion

If you have any doubts about the diagnosis, or about the recommended treatment, feel free to seek a second opinion. You are entitled to evaluate all your options, and no competent healthcare provider will object to your listening to another viewpoint.

Changing Doctors

Sometimes you may find that you are not getting along with one of the physicians treating you. The physician may seem abrupt, aloof, and uncaring, or fails to convince you of his competence. If this creates a barrier, let the physician know you wish to see someone else. The physician is probably as aware as you that a relationship based on trust and open communication has not been established, and will be happy to transfer your records to another practitioner.

But remember, a decision to change physicians should be based on reality and not on a quest to find a doctor who will promise a cure, or guarantee to relieve all your fears.

GATHERING INFORMATION

When a woman hears that she has breast cancer, her first response may be a desire to have treatment — any treatment — immediately. But breast cancer is not a medical emergency like a heart attack or an appendicitis. By the time the tumor is found, it may have been growing for years. It will not

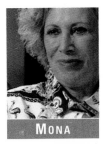

MONA

Too many doctors do not give their patients enough time. If you are not totally content with your physician, go and find somebody who will listen to you, answer your questions, and make you feel you are an important patient. A woman should be assertive and speak up, and if she wants to know why and when and where, she's entitled to these answers.

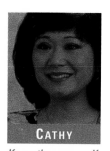

CATHY

Know thy enemy. Know what you're facing and most of your fears will become manageable. That was the most important thing to me — to educate myself about breast cancer.

QUESTIONS TO ASK YOUR DOCTOR

☐ Do you, or your clinic or hospital, have a resource center? A library?

☐ Can you refer me to breast cancer groups or organizations in this area?

☐ Where can I find more information about breast cancer?

adversely affect your outcome if you take a few weeks to organize your thoughts, gather information, and make a decision about treatment, without jeopardizing the outcome. Becoming well informed about breast cancer and about your options is one of the most important steps you can take at this stage. Knowledge of the facts will give you a sense of comfort and control.

Studies have shown that a woman's degree of satisfaction with the outcome of her treatment had to do less with the results of the treatment, and more with how much information she had when she made the decision. Take your time to gather all the facts you need, so that you can be comfortable with the decisions that will affect the rest of your life.

Your main source of information will be the professionals caring for you. Make lists of topics you want to discuss, and don't hesitate to ask any question, no matter how simple it may seem. Ask your support person to accompany you to the medical appointments, so that you have someone to help you take notes, tape record what was said, or ask additional questions.

Many medical facilities have patient resource centers where you will find collections of books, videos, and CD-ROMs on various aspects of breast cancer treatment, as well as a facilitator who can assist you.

On a regional or national level, there are several organizations that can be valuable sources of information: The American Cancer Society, The National Association of Breast Cancer Organizations (NABCO), The Susan G. Komen Breast Cancer Foundation, The Women's Information Network Against Breast Cancer (WIN-ABC), and Y-ME. These organizations and many others can be found in the Resources section at the end of the book.

The specialists at these organizations, many of whom are breast cancer survivors themselves, can answer many general questions about cancer, or send you written materials and information.

PLANNING YOUR TREATMENT

With today's early detection and improved treatment techniques, we can treat breast cancer more successfully than ever before. The following overview is intended to give you a general idea of the treatments available, and of the decision steps involved. Don't worry if you feel initially confused by the new words and concepts presented here. Most people do, at first. This information will make it easier for you to understand your physician's recommendations, and arrive at a decision.

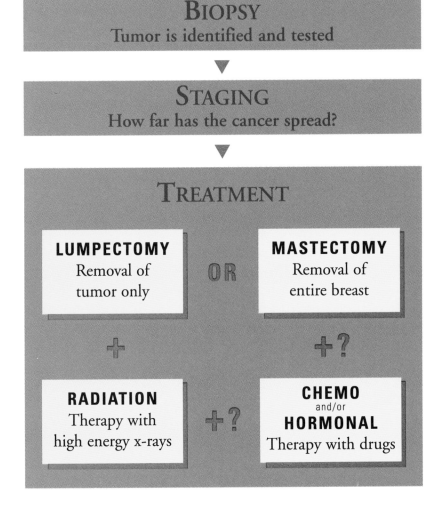

BIOPSY
Tumor is identified and tested

▼

STAGING
How far has the cancer spread?

▼

TREATMENT

LUMPECTOMY
Removal of tumor only

OR

MASTECTOMY
Removal of entire breast

+

+?

RADIATION
Therapy with high energy x-rays

+?

CHEMO
and/or
HORMONAL
Therapy with drugs

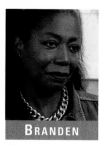

BRANDEN

Develop a really good working relationship with the physicians who are treating you, and let your feelings be known. This is your time. Make sure that everybody is on your team, and don't be afraid to speak up for yourself.

Planning your treatment should involve the entire team of specialists who consulted on your case, as well as your partner or your loved ones.

As your case progresses, your team of healthcare professionals will review the information available, and discuss your case with you and among themselves. You'll probably meet with various team members several times, while they develop a recommendation for a course of treatment that's best suited to your case.

The key thing to remember is that it is you who will make the final decision, and all the members of the team need to respect it. That's why it is so important for you to learn all you can about your disease. The more information you can gather before you begin treatment, the better you will feel about your decision, and the more active role you'll be able to take.

CHAPTER 2

Breast Cancer Basics

BREAST ANATOMY AND FUNCTION

Although the general shape of a breast is circular or tear-drop, breast tissue can be found from the collar bone to the bra line, and from the breast bone to the armpit. That is why it is important for you to examine that entire area during breast self examination, and for the surgeon to make a wide enough incision during a mastectomy.

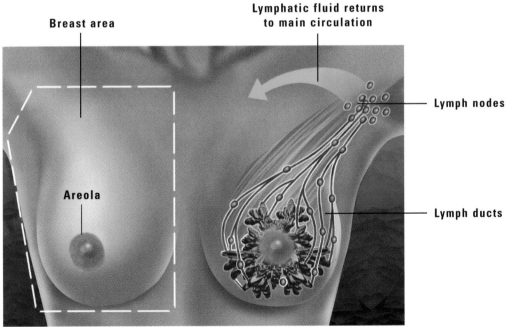

Anatomy of the breast area

Microscopic views

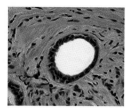

Duct, magnified x200

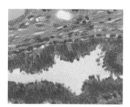

Lobe, magnified x200

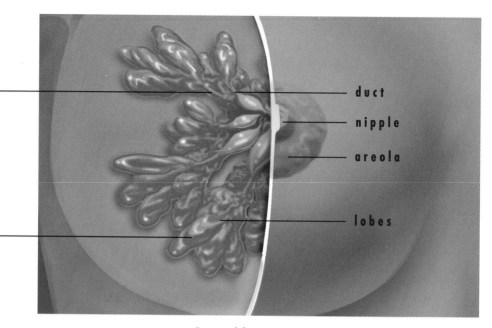

duct

nipple

areola

lobes

Internal breast structures

Breasts are made up of milk-producing glands and milk-carrying ducts, imbedded in fatty tissue and fibrous supportive tissue. The glands are grouped in sections, called *lobes*. Each lobe has many smaller *lobules* which end in dozens of tiny grape-like bulbs where milk is produced. That is why breasts usually feel lumpy to the touch. Slender tubes called *ducts* carry the milk from the lobes to the nipple.

Two muscles, the *pectoralis major* and the *pectoralis minor*, are attached to the ribs under the breast. There are no muscles within the breast itself.

Arteries and veins carry blood to and from the breast, supplying it with nutrients and oxygen. *Lymph ducts* collect *lymph* (the fluid that leaks out of the blood vessels and accumulates between cells) and bring it back into the main circulation. Along the way, lymphatic fluid is filtered through small bean-shaped organs called *lymph nodes*.

Most of the lymphatic fluid from the breast drains toward the armpit area (the *axilla*), where it is filtered through the *axillary lymph nodes*.

How Breasts Grow and Change

From birth to old age, breasts go through more changes than almost any other organ in the body.

One to two years before menarche (the first menstrual period) breasts begin to grow under the influence of the female hormones estrogen and progesterone.

During reproductive years, variations in the levels of these hormones cause the breasts to go through monthly cycles: milk glands become engorged and the breasts swell, as if getting ready for a pregnancy, then return to their inactive state again.

At menopause, levels of hormones drop, many milk producing glands shrink and disappear, and some of the breast tissue is replaced with fat.

All these changes sometimes damage the cells' DNA — the genetic material that tells the cell how to divide and grow. This damage may lead to cancer.

WHAT IS BREAST CANCER?

All organs in the body are made of cells. Individual cells are so small, they can be seen only through a microscope. Normally, cells divide in an orderly fashion to replace cells that have aged and died. Controls within each cell tell it to stop dividing if no new cells are needed.

Occasionally, damage to DNA during cell duplication may cause the controls to malfunction. Cells begin to divide uncontrollably, forming lumps or tumors.

Tumors

The word "tumor" comes from a Latin word that means "swelling." A tumor could be composed of cells that divide excessively, but do not invade or damage other parts of the body. A good example is a fibroid in the uterus, or a fibroadenoma in the breast. Both of these are called *benign*, that is, non-cancerous tumors.

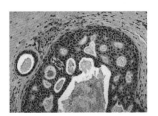

Microscopic view of cancer

Malignant tumors are composed of aggressively dividing cells that destroy surrounding tissues or travel to other parts of the body. The word "tumor" usually refers to a malignant condition, or cancer.

Growth Rate

Growth rate is the speed at which a lump or tumor grows. Different types of breast cancer grow at different rates. The time it takes for a tumor to become twice as large is called doubling time. The average *doubling time* for most breast cancer tumors is in the range of 50 to 200 days.

The change of the first normal cell into a malignant cell happens years before any evidence of cancer can be detected. It may take five to ten years for a group of abnormal cells to become large enough to be felt by hand.

Risk Factors

Who can get breast cancer? All women are at risk for developing breast cancer. It is the most common cancer in women, with about 185,000 new cases being diagnosed every year. Breast cancer also occurs in men, but very rarely.

The main risk factor for developing breast cancer is age. The older you are, the greater your chances of developing the disease. Four out of five breast cancers are found in women over the age of fifty.

A positive family history — in other words, having a first degree relative such as a mother, sister, or daughter who had breast cancer, particularly before menopause — indicates that a woman may have an increased risk of breast cancer. However, only about one in twenty cases of breast cancer is truly hereditary — that is, runs in the family. Women with breast cancer should suggest to their close female relatives that they consult their physicians about their own risk factors, and begin an effective program of early detection.

There appears to be a connection between breast cancer and estrogen. Interruptions in the levels of this hormone, such as occur during pregnancy and lactation, seem to have a protective effect. That is probably why women who had one or more children by the age of thirty are at a lower risk, while women who had an early menarche (first menstrual period) or a late menopause (last period) are at a higher risk.

Use of birth control pills has not been conclusively linked to breast cancer.

We don't know exactly what causes breast cancer, but we do know that it's probably not caused by a blow or physical injury, and that it is definitely not contagious. Recent studies show that exercise and a low fat diet may have a protective effect, while excessive alcohol intake (more than an average of one drink per day) may increase the risk.

Breast Cancer Genes

A recent well-publicized development is the discovery of the BRCA1 and BRCA2 genes.

Genes are specific areas on chromosomes that program the cell with information for growth and function. Scientists found that damage to specific genes on Chromosome 17 correlates with an increased incidence of hereditary-type breast cancer.

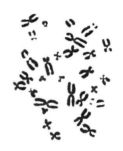

Chromosomes contain genetic information

There are tests that can detect damage to the BRCA1 and BRCA2 gene. But widespread use of this test to identify women at high risk is being debated because the benefits and consequences of knowing the results are not clear. For example, a "negative" gene test does not mean that the gene is normal. Rather, it indicates that a mutation has not been found. A negative test does not guarantee that the woman will not get breast cancer.

Conversely, a "positive" test does not mean a woman will develop breast cancer, but it does open the door to a variety of problems if the woman's insurance company or employer were to obtain this information.

The best advice for a woman with breast cancer is to suggest to her relatives that they consult a qualified risk counselor before undergoing any genetic testing.

Types of Breast Cancer

The most common forms of breast cancer come from cells that line the milk ducts (ductal cancer) or the milk-producing lobules (lobular cancer).

In the early stages, cancer cells divide locally, and do not cross the wall of the duct or lobule. This type of cancer is called *in situ* — meaning "in place." Today 15% to 20% of breast cancers fall into the *in situ* category — either ductal carcinoma *in situ* (DCIS) or lobular carcinoma *in situ* (LCIS).

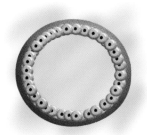

Normal duct

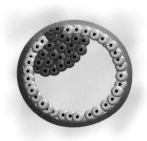

In situ cancer

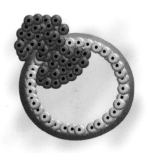

Invasive cancer

DCIS cancers are highly curable. Some authorities don't even refer to them as cancer, but rather as "precancerous lesions," since DCIS may never progress to be an invasive cancer.

LCIS is a non-invasive growth that is not considered cancerous, but women who are diagnosed with LCIS have about a 1% per year risk of developing invasive breast cancer. Twenty years after diagnosis, this risk is about 18%. What is interesting is that the invasive cancer can occur in either breast, and not necessarily where the LCIS was originally found.

More advanced than *in situ* cancers are infiltrating cancers where malignant cells cross the lining of the duct or lobule, and begin to invade, or infiltrate, adjacent tissues. The most common type of breast cancer is the infiltrating ductal carcinoma. More than half of all cases are this type.

Other types of breast cancer are less common. Two examples are *Paget's Disease*, a cancerous growth that first appears as scaling on the nipple, and *inflammatory cancer*, a rare form of cancer that grows quickly, causing redness and swelling of the breast.

How Cancer Spreads

As a malignant tumor grows, it may spread locally, invading and sometimes destroying other tissues, or cells may break away from the tumor and get into the lymphatic vessels. Some of the breakaway cells will be trapped in the lymph nodes of the armpit, or axilla. Examination of these nodes by a procedure called axillary lymph node dissection can help determine the stage, or degree of spread, of the cancer.

If cancer cells escape beyond the lymph nodes, or enter the circulatory system directly, they can spread to the liver, brain, lungs, and bones, forming new tumors, called *metastases*. These distant metastases are the most worrisome, because they can damage vital organs. This advanced stage of breast cancer, called *metastatic* cancer, is less common and its management is more difficult.

To make sure that no cancer cells remain anywhere in the body, it is often necessary to use systemic therapy — therapy that reaches all the organs, in all parts of the body. This is explained in the Chemotherapy and Hormonal Therapy chapters.

CHAPTER 3

Diagnosis & Staging

The only sure way to confirm a diagnosis of breast cancer is to perform a biopsy — that is, to remove a small piece of the tumor, and have it examined under a microscope by a pathologist — a specialist in tumor identification.

The sample can be obtained either with a needle, or surgically. Odds are that if you are reading this book, you already may have had a biopsy that showed your tumor was malignant. If so, feel free to skip to the Staging section on page 31.

BIOPSY

If the tumor is small, or if there is a good possibility that it is not cancerous, your physician may choose either a *fine needle aspiration* or a *core needle biopsy*.

Fine Needle Aspiration

Fine Needle Aspiration, or FNA, is done with a very thin needle connected to a syringe. The needle is moved in and out several times to obtain the best sample possible.

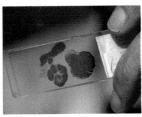

Tumor sample ready for examination under microscope

The material drawn into the syringe will be sent to a pathologist for analysis. Even if no cancer cells are found, your doctor may want to have the lump removed surgically.

Core Needle Biopsy

Core Needle Biopsy is done with a larger needle, which can yield a larger sample. The procedure can be done under a local anesthetic and takes only a few minutes. Most women who have had the procedure report only minor discomfort.

If the lesion is non-palpable (in other words, cannot be felt by hand) the core needle biopsy can be done using special mammography equipment (called a stereotactic unit). This equipment enables the physician to place the needle precisely into the tumor, even if it is as small as a pea. The biopsy also can be done using ultrasound equipment. The choice generally depends on what your physician is most comfortable with.

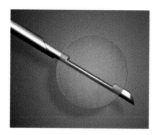

*Core needle taking
a biopsy sample*

The core biopsy itself is performed with a device that works like an ear-piercing instrument: it propels a needle very rapidly through the lesion. A special notch in the needle traps a sliver of tissue for examination. Samples obtained with core biopsy are large enough to be cut into thin slices and examined under the microscope, providing a diagnosis that some doctors feel is more reliable than that from a FNA.

Mammotome Biopsy

This device uses a needle with a vacuum assist to obtain a much larger sample. Unlike open surgical biopsy, with requires a skin incision, or core biopsy, which requires multiple insertions of the device, the Mammotome Breast Biopsy system needs only a single insertion done under local anesthesia.

Surgical Biopsy

Another way your doctor may choose to obtain a biopsy is surgically. A surgical biopsy is performed under local or general anesthesia. Most surgical biopsies are excisional, in other words the surgeon removes (excises) the entire tumor.

The surgical biopsy takes about an hour, and causes minimal post-operative pain that goes away in a few days. You can usually begin doing non-strenuous work the day after the biopsy, although you should not lift heavy objects for a few weeks. The incision usually heals within ten days.

TUMOR TESTING

The sample of tumor will be examined under a microscope by a pathologist, who will identify the cells and determine whether the tumor is benign or malignant.

If the tumor is malignant, additional tests may be performed to help your physician determine the type of treatment that will be most effective.

Estrogen Receptors and Progesterone Receptors

One of the most common tests is for estrogen and progesterone receptors. *Receptors* are areas on the surface of cells to which substances, such as the hormones *estrogen* and *progesterone*, can bind — much like a lock accepts a key. When the hormone binds to its receptor, it activates the cell, making it divide.

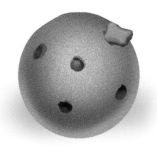

Estrogen binding to receptor site

If a tumor is composed of cells that have estrogen or progesterone receptors, it is called *estrogen receptor positive*, or *progesterone receptor positive*, or *hormone receptor positive*. Such tumors can be treated with drugs that block the action of the hormones. Tumors lacking estrogen and progesterone receptors usually can not be treated with hormonal therapy.

HER-2/neu (c-erb B2)

An *oncogene* is a gene which when turned on, leads to development of a cancer. Women with abnormally high levels of an oncogene called Her-2/neu tend to develop much more aggressive breast cancer. A new technique, the HercepTest, can determine your level of HER-2/neu and help your oncologist decide if you are a good candidate for a new antibody called Herceptin.

Other Tumor Characteristics

There are other factors, which are currently being evaluated, that may help determine the tumor's response, but most are still considered to be unproven: *Percent S-phase, Ploidy,* and *p53.*

Percent (%) S-phase

When cells divide, they go through a number of specific steps, or phases. S-phase is the phase of the cell cycle in which DNA is replicating -- making copies of itself, so that a complete set will go to each new cell. Having a high percentage of cells in the S-phase indicates more rapid tumor growth.

Ploidy

Genes are clusters of DNA that are strung together in long strands called chromosomes, and form the "blue-prints" that determine what a cell does and how it works. Cells having an abnormal number of chromosomes (or an abnormal amount of DNA) are called aneuploid and may indicate a somewhat worse prognosis.

p53

A *suppressor gene* is a gene which protects the body against cancer. If this gene is mutated (damaged), its protective effect may be lost. Mutated p53 can be detected in the cells of some breast cancers and is associated with poorer prognosis.

THE PATHOLOGY REPORT

If you had a fine needle aspiration, the pathologist may be able to identify the general type of cancer and report within an hour. A larger sample, such as from a core needle biopsy or surgical biopsy, is required for a more complete identification and diagnosis. This report will generally take several days. Depending on the results, the surgeon may decide to enlarge the area of tissue removed, or to perform an axillary lymph node dissection — that is, to examine the lymph nodes in the armpit to check for possible cancer spread. This procedure is described in detail in Chapter 4.

The final pathology report will specify the size of the tumor, what type of cell the tumor is composed of, and how aggressive the cells are — in other words, how rapidly and energetically they seem to be growing and dividing. This information is essential for planning your treatment.

ADDITIONAL TESTS

Why more tests? The biopsy will confirm the diagnosis of cancer, but it will not show whether the cancer has spread to other parts of the body.

To find this out, additional tests may need to be performed, including chest x-rays, blood tests, CTs or MRIs of the abdomen or other parts of the body, and bone scans. This information is important to determine the stage of the tumor.

CAT scan, CT scan, or Computerized Axial Tomography all mean the same thing. This test uses ordinary x-rays, and a rotating film/source system to obtain detailed images of your body. The test is painless and takes less than an hour.

MRI or Magnetic Resonance Imaging uses a combination of magnetic energy and ordinary radio waves to create images of the inside of your body. Because the MRI unit can feel cramped, notify the technologist or your physician if you feel uncomfortable in confined spaces. MRI is painless, and does not expose you to x-ray radiation. The test takes about an hour.

Some of the more common sites to which breast cancer cells may metastasize, or spread, include bones. The most effective way to find these metastases is to perform a *nuclear bone scan*. This test is generally done if the tumor is large, or the lymph nodes are positive and there is a good chance that tumor cells may be found in other areas of the body. For this scan, tiny amounts of radioactive substance are injected into a vein. Once inside the body, the radioactive substance concentrates in areas where there is an unusually increased number of blood vessels — a "hot spot" — that may correspond to a new growth of cancer cells.

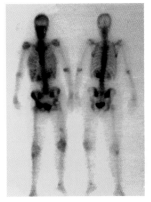

Bone scan

STAGING

How Stage is Determined

Each cancer is unique, each woman is different, and the combination of treatment options is practically endless. To help determine who should get what treatment, cancer specialists rely on *staging* — a system that places the cancer into a certain group. The stage of your tumor is the most important factor in deciding what type of treatment is best for you.

TNM

In simplified form, staging is based on: the *size* of the tumor; presence of cancer cells in the *lymph nodes*; and *metastasis*, or spread, to other organs. This is the so called TNM — tumor, node, metastasis — staging system.

Tumor size is determined when the tumor is removed and sent to the pathologist. **Lymph nodes** are checked for evidence of tumor spread at the time of surgery in a procedure called axillary lymph node dissection. **Metastasis**, or spread to other organs, is assessed with bone scans, x-rays, CAT scans, and blood tests.

Putting all this information together is called **staging**.

Stages of Breast Cancer
There are several staging systems in use today. Here is one of them:

Stage 0 (*in situ*)**:**
Ductal or lobular carcinoma *in situ,* or Paget's Disease of the nipple.

Tumors, actual size

1 cm

Stage I:
Tumor is 2 cm (3/4 inch) or smaller. Axillary lymph nodes are negative and there is no evidence of distant metastases.

Stage II:
Tumor is 2-5 cm in size (about 3/4 to 2 inches). Axillary lymph nodes may or may not be positive for cancer. Even if the tumor is smaller than 2 cm, but the lymph nodes are positive, cancer is still considered Stage II.

Stage III:
Tumor is larger than 5 cm (2 inches) and axillary lymph nodes are positive. Tumor may extend into the pectoral muscles or into the skin of the breast, but there are no distant metastases.

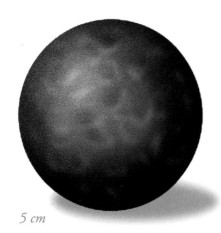

2 cm

Stage IV:
If metastasis to other organs has occurred, cancer is considered Stage IV regardless of the size of the tumor, or the number of positive axillary lymph nodes.

You may find it helpful to think of stage as degree of risk presented by a particular tumor.

Very tiny tumors that have not spread to lymph nodes, present a lower risk, and may be managed with breast conserving surgical removal of the tumor plus a course of radiation therapy, and perhaps a less aggressive form of hormonal therapy or chemotherapy.

5 cm

Slightly larger tumors, still smaller than about a half inch (1 cm) and still without evidence of lymph node spread, may need more aggressive chemotherapy.

For larger, high-risk tumors that have invaded the lymph nodes there are a wide variety of options, including combination chemotherapy and high dose chemotherapy with bone marrow transplant.

CHAPTER 4

Surgery

In treating breast cancer, radiation therapy, chemotherapy, or hormonal therapy cannot replace surgery. To ensure the best chance for successful treatment, it is important first to remove as much of the tumor as possible, using the most direct approach possible. That means some type of surgery.

Today there are two surgical options:

One is to remove just the tumor with a safety margin of healthy breast tissue around it, conserving most of the breast. This is called *wide local excision, partial mastectomy,* or *lumpectomy.* This *breast-conserving surgery* is usually followed by *radiation therapy* — treatment of the breast area with high energy x-rays to destroy any cancer cells that may have remained in the breast area.

The other option is to remove the entire breast, which is called a *mastectomy.* In the past, women dreaded this operation almost as much as the cancer itself. But the mastectomy techniques used today are much less disfiguring than the ones used in years past, and offer better possibilities for cosmetic reconstruction.

Many studies have now proven that breast-conserving therapy is as effective as a mastectomy. The choice depends on the type, size, and degree of spread of your tumor, and on your personal preference.

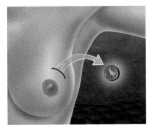

LUMPECTOMY
removal of the tumor with a margin of healthy tissue.

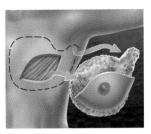

MASTECTOMY
removal of the entire breast.

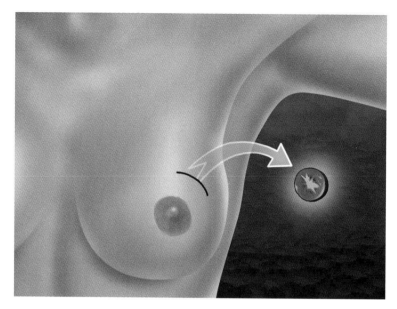

QUESTIONS TO ASK
YOUR SURGEON:

☐ Is lumpectomy an
option for me? Why or
why not?

☐ How much breast tis-
sue will be removed?

☐ How will my breast
look after the treat-
ment? Can you show
me pictures?

☐ Where, and how big
will the scar be?

☐ How much pain should
I expect in the first few
days after the proce-
dure?

☐ Do I need to arrange to
have someone come
help me with daily
activities?

☐ How long before I can
go back to my regular
work or leisure activi-
ties?

☐ Will there be any long
term effects?

LUMPECTOMY

What is a Lumpectomy?

If the tumor is small and confined to a single location in the breast, you may have the option of having breast-conserving surgery. The goal of this relatively simple procedure is to remove the whole tumor, while conserving as much breast tissue as possible. A margin of normal breast tissue is also removed to make sure no malignant cells are left behind.

The technical term for this type of surgery is *partial mastectomy*. Most people commonly refer to it as a *lumpectomy* — a "lump-removal" so to speak. This term is somewhat misleading, since a margin of normal tissue must also be removed. Depending on how much breast tissue is removed, the procedure may also be called *wide excision, segmental mastectomy*, or *quadrantectomy*. The specific technique used may vary from surgeon to surgeon and from case to case.

The cosmetic result of breast conserving surgery will vary with the location and size of the tumor, and the size of the breast. Removing a large tumor from a large breast may result in a normal-looking breast, but removing even a small tumor from a small breast may lead to noticeable change in breast size and shape, and perhaps a cosmetically unacceptable result.

A few very large tumors may be treated first with chemotherapy or radiation in order to shrink them before being removed surgically.

Breast conserving surgery almost always requires additional treatment of the breast area with high energy x-rays (radiation therapy) to reduce the chance that any surviving cancer cells are left behind.

Before Surgery

If your tumor was found on a mammogram, but is difficult or impossible to feel by touch, your surgeon may request that a *needle localization* procedure be done before you go to surgery. For this procedure a radiologist will use a special mammography unit to pinpoint the location of the tumor, then mark it by inserting a thin wire into the breast. The surgeon will follow this wire to find the tumor more easily during surgery.

A lumpectomy may be done in a hospital operating room, or in an outpatient surgery center. You may be able to go home the same day. You may want to have a friend or relative accompany you to the hospital, to provide moral support, to meet you after surgery, and to drive you home.

Before the surgery you'll meet with the anesthesiologist to decide whether you'll have general or local anesthesia. The choice depends on your health and on your personal preferences.

You'll also be asked to sign an informed consent form as an indication that you understand the procedure and the possible complications, such as infection and bleeding. Make sure to read the form carefully and ask for explanations of any parts that you are not comfortable with.

The Surgical Procedure

A lumpectomy takes about an hour. The surgeon will make a skin incision over the tumor area and remove the tumor, with a small amount of surrounding healthy breast tissue. This margin, about one-half to three-quarters of an inch in thickness, helps decrease the chances that any tumor cells are left behind.

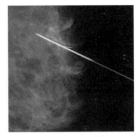

Breast needle localization x-ray

QUESTIONS TO ASK YOUR ANESTHESIOLOGIST:

☐ **If I have general anesthesia, how long will it take me to get back to normal?**

☐ **What will I feel and hear if I have local anesthesia?**

☐ **Will you give me something to control the pain after I wake up from the anesthetic?**

The surgical specimen will be sent to a pathologist who will examine it under a microscope and determine whether the margins were clear of tumor cells. If tumor cells are found along the edges (*dirty margins*), it means that some cancerous cells may have been left behind. Another lumpectomy may be done to get *clear margins*. In some cases, a mastectomy may be required.

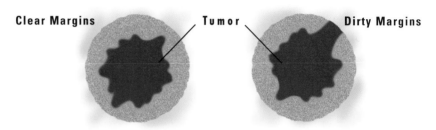

Clear Margins   **Tumor**   **Dirty Margins**

Breast tissue removed during lumpectomy

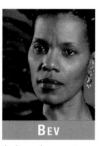

BEV

I chose lumpectomy. When surgery took place, they found out that the edges were not clear of tumor. When I came out from under the medication that night, I signed another paper for them to go on and do the mastectomy the next day.

Recovery after Lumpectomy

After the lumpectomy, you'll be taken to the recovery room for a short while, and then discharged to go home.

If you didn't have an axillary lymph node dissection at the same time as the lumpectomy, you'll be able to resume normal activities almost immediately.

Follow the aftercare instructions you receive regarding how long to keep the incision dry, when to return for a follow up visit to your surgeon, and when to have the sutures removed.

Radiation Therapy

An important part of breast-conserving treatment is radiation therapy. Radiation therapy uses high energy x-rays aimed at the breast area to kill any possible remaining cancer cells. This involves treatments five days a week for five to seven weeks at a special facility. Each session takes just a few minutes.

You can learn more about radiation therapy in Chapter 6.

Is Lumpectomy Right for Me?

What is better, mastectomy or lumpectomy? Numerous research studies, involving thousands of women and many years of follow up, show that there is no difference in survival between the two procedures.

Besides being equally effective, breast-conserving surgery offers several advantages over a mastectomy. You keep your breast, (although you may notice a change in shape), and you avoid the emotional trauma of losing the breast. Sensation in the nipple and skin area can be preserved, and a good cosmetic result can be expected.

However, not all women can have breast-conserving surgery. A lumpectomy would not be recommended in the following situations:

- There is more than one tumor in the breast.
- The tumor is so large or the breast so small that the cosmetic result would not be satisfactory after removal of the tumor.
- The tumor was found to extend beyond the margins of the tissue removed during initial surgery.
- You are not willing to have radiation therapy, or there is no convenient radiation therapy facility near you.
- You prefer to have a mastectomy, for peace of mind or other reasons.

It is important to remember that no decision needs to be made overnight. You can take up to several weeks to gather information. You do not need to make the decision alone. Consult your healthcare professionals, and consider getting a second opinion.

The American Cancer Society's Reach to Recovery program, WIN-ABC's Breast Buddy program, the Susan G. Komen Foundation, and other organizations can put you in touch with other women who had the same type of surgery that you are considering, and will be happy to discuss your choice with you.

See the Resources section for more information on these organizations.

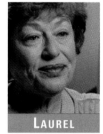

LAUREL

I had a lumpectomy with a local anesthetic. It was extremely easy and when it was over I felt physically very good. I was able to go home with relatively little pain.

ADVANTAGES OF LUMPECTOMY:

- as effective as mastectomy
- breast is spared
- preserves normal nipple and skin sensation
- yields good cosmetic results

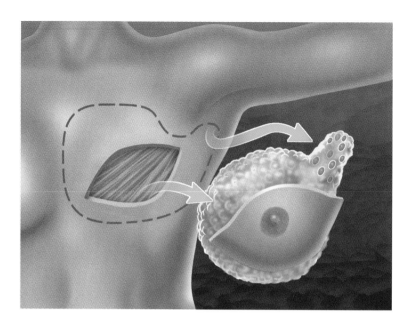

MASTECTOMY

The other option for surgical treatment of breast cancer is mastectomy.

What is a Mastectomy?

Mastectomy, or surgical removal of the breast, has been used to treat breast cancer for over a century.

The radical mastectomy, which removed the entire breast, the lymph nodes in the armpit, and one of the major muscles of the chest wall, was based on the assumption that the more tissue removed, the better the chances of curing the cancer. This procedure caused so much deformity, that women feared it as much as the cancer itself.

In the 1970's and 1980's, research proved that there was no advantage in removing the chest muscles, and the *modified radical mastectomy*, which spares these muscles yielding a more cosmetically acceptable result, was introduced. Now the radical mastectomy is almost never performed.

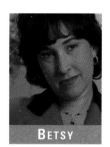

BETSY

The tumor was three and half centimeters, and it encompassed part of the nipple area. The doctors explained to me that I would have to have the nipple removed and a large portion of the breast, even if I had a lumpectomy. My breasts aren't that large, so I opted for a mastectomy and breast reconstruction.

Today's modified radical mastectomy removes as much of the breast tissue as possible, including the nipple and areola, and a number of axillary lymph nodes, but not the muscles. Patients can choose from a variety of reconstruction techniques that offer pleasing cosmetic results.

Before Surgery

A mastectomy is generally done in a hospital, under general anesthesia. After a date is set, someone on your surgeon's staff will review with you the admission process for the particular hospital where the operation will take place.

Ask someone in the surgeon's or hospital's business office whether your insurance covers surgical fees, hospital room, anesthesiologist's fees, and other charges.

Make a list of all the medications you are taking, both prescription and over-the-counter, since some of them may have adverse effects during anesthesia or surgery. (For example, aspirin-containing preparations can increase bleeding.) Some medications may need to be discontinued weeks before surgery.

Pack all the personal belongings you may need.

Decide if you want someone to accompany you to the hospital. Most people undergoing surgery enjoy having a friend or relative meet them after the procedure.

You'll be instructed not to eat or drink anything after midnight on the night before the surgery.

On the day of the surgery, you'll first go through an admission process at the hospital. Your surgeon already will have reviewed with you all aspects of the procedure, and the possible risks and complications. On the day of admission, the hospital staff will ask you to sign an *informed consent form* listing your doctor's name and the name of the surgical procedure you are having. An informed consent form requires that you verify the following:

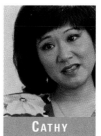

CATHY

I knew that my surgery was just a few days away, and I looked down at my body and at this right breast and I said, "I'm very proud of you. You're beautiful. But I am very sorry, you have to go. So goodbye." It was necessary. I'm glad that I made my peace with it.

THINGS TO TAKE WITH YOU TO THE HOSPITAL:

- nightgown
- slippers
- toiletries
- books
- Walkman
- favorite pillow
- change of loose clothing for when you go home

- The risks of the surgery and the anesthetic have been explained to you
- Medications, anesthesia, and blood transfusions, may be administered
- Any tissue removed may be examined and disposed of
- You understand all of the foregoing and consent to the surgery.

Make sure you feel comfortable with what you are signing. Cross out and initial anything you don't agree to. If there is anything on the form that worries you, ask to see your doctor.

Blood transfusions are rarely needed during lumpectomies or mastectomies, but may be required for certain types of breast reconstruction. You may wish to discuss with your physician the possibility of donating and storing your own blood before your surgery so that it can be used, should you need it.

QUESTIONS TO ASK YOUR ANESTHESIOLOGIST:

☐ Will you give me something to help me relax before surgery?

☐ How long will it take me to get back to normal after a general anesthetic?

☐ What are the side effects of anesthesia?

An anesthesiologist or a nurse anesthetist will meet with you and select a general anesthetic that is best suited to your medical condition. They need to know about:

- Your medical history and any problems with your heart, lungs, or circulation.
- Any current conditions such as skin infections, colds, or tooth decay.
- Any allergies.
- Your smoking and drinking patterns.
- Any prescriptions, over-the-counter medications, or drugs that you may be taking.

The Surgical Procedure

The anesthesiologist will meet you in the staging area, start an intravenous line (an "IV") in one of your arms using a small needle, and perhaps give you something to help you relax.

When the surgical team is ready, you will be taken to the operating room. Several devices will be attached to you, such as an automatic blood pressure cuff, a heart monitor, and a blood oxygen monitor. The anesthesiologist will inject a drug into your vein through the tubing, and you will fall asleep almost immediately. A tube may be placed in your throat to maintain a clear way for you to breathe during the surgery. Your blood pressure, pulse, and breathing will be closely monitored during the entire procedure.

The total mastectomy takes two to three hours. Breast tissue extends from the collar bone to the edge of the ribs, and from the breast bone to the muscles in the back of the armpit. The surgeon will make an elliptical incision to separate the breast from the chest wall, then remove as much of the breast tissue as possible.

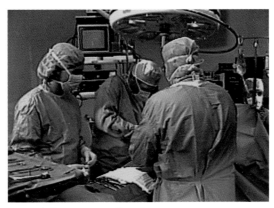

Surgeons performing a mastectomy

The tissue will be sent to the pathologist, who will examine it for any evidence of cancer spread beyond the breast.

Unless your tumor was very small, you also may have an axillary lymph node dissection — removal of a number of lymph nodes from your armpit for examination by the pathologist. Presence or absence of cancer cells in these lymph nodes will help determine your future treatments.

You will find more information about this procedure in the section on axillary lymph node dissection later in this chapter.

If you've decided to have immediate reconstruction of the breast, the plastic surgeon will take over while you are still asleep. Reconstruction can be done using your own tissues — from the abdomen, back, or buttocks, or using a synthetic implant. The procedure may take anywhere from an hour, to six or eight hours, depending on the method used. You can learn about reconstruction options in more detail in Chapter 5.

When the procedure (mastectomy or node dissection) is completed, one or two tubes called *drains* will be placed under the skin to help drain the fluid that accumulates at the site of surgery. If you go home with the drains, you'll receive instructions on how to care for them.

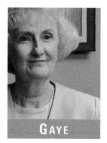

GAYE

I was not happy about having to deal with drains. The nurse showed me how to use them, and I said, "I don't think I can do this." But I did, and my husband helped me. He was right there with everything that we did.

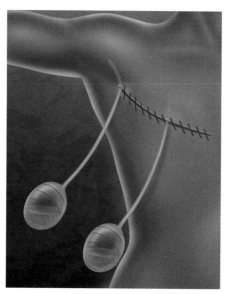

You will be given specific instructions on how to manage your drains. Generally, after washing your hands, you will disconnect the suction bulb from the drain itself, check and write down the color and volume of fluid, discard the fluid, squeeze the drain bulb, and keeping it squeezed, reattach it to the drain. The bulb will not re-expand right away, but will apply a gentle suction to the drain to help remove the fluid. The drains will be removed after the drainage slows — usually within five to ten days.

Recovery after Mastectomy

After surgery, you'll be taken to the recovery room. As you wake up from the anesthetic, you may feel cold, and your throat may be sore from the tube used for anesthesia. You may fade between waking and sleeping for several hours.

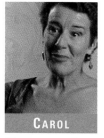

CAROL

I have a very clear memory of the first time I took the bandages off. I literally went crazy. All of a sudden it was in my face. That breast wasn't there anymore. And it wouldn't ever be there.

Whatever surgery they are going to have, most women like to have a friend or relative meet them after the operation. You can ask your surgeon how long it will take before you will be brought to your room after surgery and to arrange with the hospital to allow that person to meet you there.

Most women will stay in the hospital for one or two nights after a mastectomy, and somewhat longer after a mastectomy with reconstruction.

Each woman reacts to surgery differently. Many can take a short walk in and out of their hospital room the day of surgery. The next day, most are able to eat a regular diet and get around.

Once you're home, you'll probably feel more tired than usual for a while. Don't be discouraged. You've just been through general anesthesia and major surgery, and fatigue is to be expected.

Take sponge baths for a few days after surgery until your incision starts to heal. Don't shower until your drains are removed, and then do so gently and pat, rather than rub, the incision.

Immediately after surgery, you'll probably have trouble moving your arm due to muscle tightness and soreness around the shoulder. Use the arm as tolerated immediately after surgery, but avoid active stretching or pulling until the drains are removed and you get your doctor's approval. Don't be afraid to enlist the help of a friend or relative until your arm function returns.

Many women return to work as soon as they feel better, even while their chemotherapy and radiation treatments are continuing. If your job requires lifting or strenuous physical activity, you may need to change your activities until you have fully regained your strength.

If you had an axillary lymph node dissection you may experience numbness in the upper inner arm and armpit area, caused by injury to one of the nerves. If this happens to you, you may need to be particularly careful when you shave your underarm. The numbness will usually improve over months or years, but the feeling may never be completely normal.

Another side effect of axillary lymph node dissection is swelling of the arm, called lymphedema, which is caused by scarring around lymphatic ducts injured during surgery, or as a result of radiation therapy.

You can learn more about lymphedema later in this chapter.

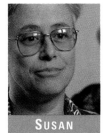

SUSAN

After surgery I got up and started moving my arms as soon as I possibly could, doing slow and gentle breathing. I think exercises are absolutely essential for having a rapid and easy recovery.

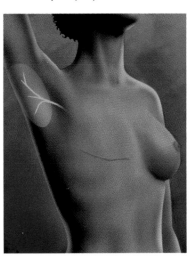

Area of numbness

QUESTIONS TO ASK YOUR SURGEON:

☐ **How much pain should I expect in the first few days after the procedure?**

☐ **What can I do to relieve the pain?**

☐ **Do I need to arrange to have someone help me with my daily activities?**

☐ **How long before I can go back to my regular work or leisure activities?**

Exercises after Mastectomy

Never attempt to begin exercising without specific instructions from your healthcare provider. Exercises must be done in stages.

After the drains are removed, your doctor or physical therapist may assign pendulum-like movements with your arm, to begin loosening any tightness in the shoulder area:

- Holding on to something for support (such as a chair or desk), lean forward at the waist and swing your arm in gradually enlarging circles. Make ten circles, rest, then repeat in the other direction.

After the sutures are removed, you may be told to begin stretching exercises to regain full motion in the shoulder:

- Walk your fingers up the wall, until you feel mild pain in the incision, and note how far you can reach each day.
- Throw a rope or an old tie over a door, and move your arms up and down in a see-saw motion.
- Walk your arm up your back as far as you can.

Many communities offer swimming, exercise, and dance classes specifically for breast cancer patients. The YWCA Encore program is one of them. Check the Resources section for other suggestions.

Is Mastectomy Right for Me?

Numerous research studies, involving thousands of women and many years of follow-up, show that there is no difference in *survival* in patients treated with lumpectomy with radiation, or with mastectomy.

It should be noted that there is a slightly higher rate of *local cancer recurrence* (in the breast area itself) following lumpectomy: one out of a hundred women treated with lumpectomy will develop a local recurrence within a year. (In other words, there is a 1% per year recurrence rate. The chance of having a recurrence within ten years is 10%.) Local recurrences are not life threatening, and can be controlled by performing a mastectomy.

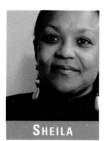

SHEILA

The clusters of cancerous cells were scattered throughout the breast, making lumpectomy not a choice. Because if they removed enough tissue the breast would be totally misshapen, and there would also be the possibility of cancer cells left behind.

Since there is no difference in numbers of life-threatening distant metastases (cancer in other sites in the body) between lumpectomy and mastectomy, there is no difference in *life expectancy* between the two procedures.

So the choice is between running a slightly higher risk of a local recurrence following lumpectomy, or accepting a mastectomy.

Remember that there is no rush to make a decision. You can take two to three weeks to review the information, and to make the decision. Consult your health-care professionals, possibly seek a second opinion, and discuss your thoughts with your loved ones.

The advantages of a mastectomy are that no radiation therapy is required, and there is a decreased risk of local recurrence. Some women prefer the procedure because of the peace of mind they expect after the removal of the breast.

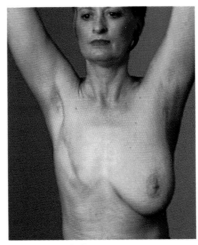

A healed mastectomy scar

QUESTIONS TO ASK YOUR DOCTOR:

- ☐ Is lumpectomy an option for me? Why or why not?
- ☐ Does a mastectomy decrease the chances of the cancer coming back?
- ☐ How will I look after a mastectomy if I decide against reconstruction?
- ☐ Can you show me pictures?
- ☐ Can you refer me to a plastic surgeon so I can discuss my reconstruction options?
- ☐ What kind of recon-struction procedure do you think would be best for me?
- ☐ Who can I talk to about my concerns about appearance, dating, pregnancy, etc?

The disadvantages include more extensive surgery, and the emotional impact of losing the entire breast, including the nipple.

Your choice will be dictated by various factors. Here are a few considerations that would favor mastectomy over lumpectomy:

- The tumor is so big or the breast so small that the cosmetic result would not be satisfactory after tumor removal.
- There is more than one tumor location in the breast.
- You are unwilling or unable to undergo radiation treatment.
- You prefer to have a mastectomy.

The American Cancer Society's Reach to Recovery program, WIN-ABC's Breast Buddy program, the Susan G. Komen Foundation, and other organizations in your area can put you in touch with other women who had the same type of surgery that you are considering, and who will be happy to discuss your choice with you. See the Resources section for information on how to contact these organizations.

AXILLARY LYMPH NODE DISSECTION

Arteries and veins carry blood to and from various parts of the body. Whatever fluid seeps out of these blood vessels is returned to the blood stream by a network of thin tubes called *lymphatic ducts*. This fluid, called *lymph*, helps the body dispose of foreign particles or other debris that can collect in the spaces between cells.

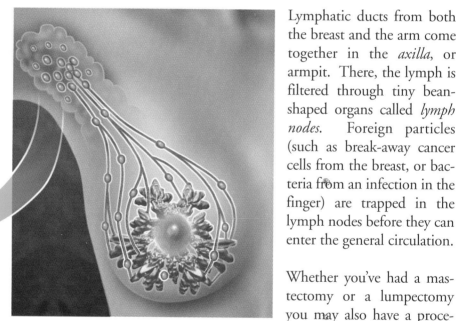

Some of the lymph nodes are removed for examination

Lymphatic ducts from both the breast and the arm come together in the *axilla*, or armpit. There, the lymph is filtered through tiny bean-shaped organs called *lymph nodes*. Foreign particles (such as break-away cancer cells from the breast, or bacteria from an infection in the finger) are trapped in the lymph nodes before they can enter the general circulation.

Whether you've had a mastectomy or a lumpectomy you may also have a procedure called *axillary lymph node dissection*. Your surgeon will remove some of the lymph nodes from your armpit and have them examined for evidence of cancer spread. Removing the lymph nodes does not help eliminate the cancer from your body. But determining whether cancer cells have spread to these lymph nodes, is important for deciding what additional therapy will be needed.

The Surgical Procedure

An axillary lymph node dissection can be done through a separate small incision in the armpit at the time of a lumpectomy, or through the main surgical incision as part of a mastectomy. The surgeon will remove a portion of the fat pad within which ten to twenty lymph nodes are imbedded. The tissue removed will be sent to the pathologist. Each node will be sliced and examined under the microscope for presence of cancer cells. The pathology report, which your physician will receive three to ten days after surgery, will indicate how many nodes were positive (in other words, had cancer cells in them).

An axillary lymph node dissection takes about an hour. The surgeon will need to exercise particular care during the dissection to avoid injuring one of several important nerves that pass through this area.

After the surgery, a drain may be placed into the armpit to help remove blood and fluid that seeps out from the operated area. Care for the incision is the same as for the lumpectomy or mastectomy: keeping it dry until the incision begins to heal and the drains are removed.

Sentinel Node Biopsy

Some centers offer a procedure called sentinel node biopsy as an alternative to axillary lymph node dissection. During surgery, a blue dye is injected around the tumor. The lymphatic fluid in that area carries the dye to the first node in its path - the sentinel node. That single node is removed and examined. If no cancer cells are found, the surgeon can assume that the other nodes are free of cancer as well. In that case, you will not need to have a full axillary lymph node dissection and will not run the risk of damage to nerves and lymph ducts that often occurs with the standard procedure.

Complications After Axillary Lymph Node Dissection

Damage to one or more of the nerves that pass through the axilla, either accidentally or because the injury was unavoidable, may result in long term numbness in the armpit area, or in weakness in some of the shoulder muscles. Often the numbness will improve over several years, but the sensitivity will never be normal. The weakness can generally be overcome with time.

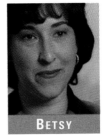

BETSY

I learned quickly that it was important to talk to doctors and nurses about not getting blood pressure taken or injections on the affected arm, to be careful when gardening, and what not. I do a lot of animal rescue and have to be careful with cat bites to the affected area.

Lymphedema

One of the more serious problems that may arise after an axillary lymph node dissection is a condition called lymphedema. It's caused by progressive scarring of lymph vessels in the underarm area after removal of the lymph nodes and their connecting ducts. The circulation of lymph fluid is slowed, causing swelling of the arm, limiting its function, and making the arm more prone to infection.

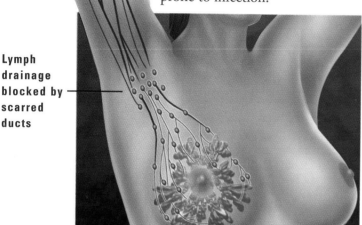

Arm swollen

Lymph drainage blocked by scarred ducts

Lymphedema

As many as 10-20% of women undergoing axillary lymph node dissection will develop lymphedema of the arm. The condition may occur soon after surgery, or years later. While it is difficult to predict who will develop lymphedema, there are several precautions that you must take to help you avoid it. These include avoiding heavy lifting, and blood tests or injuries to the arm on the side of surgery.

Precautions that will help protect your arm from lymphedema:

- Avoid sunburns, burns while cooking, and harsh chemicals.
- Have all injections, vaccinations, blood samples, and blood pressure tests done on the other arm whenever possible.
- Use an electric razor with a narrow head for underarm shaving.
- Carry heavy packages or handbags on the other arm.
- Wash cuts promptly, treat them with antibacterial medication, and cover them with a sterile bandage; check for redness or soreness.
- Never cut cuticles; use hand cream or lotion instead.
- Wear watches or jewelry loosely, if at all, on the operated arm.
- Wear protective gloves when gardening. Use a thimble if you sew.
- Use insect repellent to avoid bites and stings.
- Avoid tight elastic cuffs on blouses and nightgowns.
- If your arm becomes red, swollen, or feels hot, call your doctor at once.

EXTERNAL BREAST FORMS

Many women choose to have no reconstruction of any type after the mastectomy. Some make this decision because they want to avoid extra surgery. Others because they're comfortable with their appearance and body image.

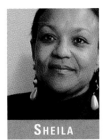

SHEILA

In the beginning, I started out with external prostheses. I didn't realize that I would end up with double D's again. These things are heavy! Wearing them eight hours gave me chest pain, backache, and headache, and so pretty soon, I began leaving them in the drawer, except when I needed to look "normal." And then I decided... "reconstruction."

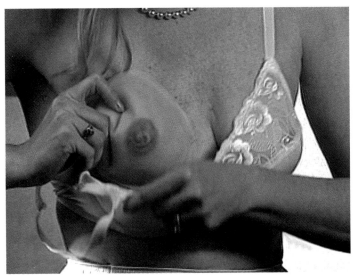

Lifelike prostheses can be custom-made

Breast forms, or *prostheses* as they are also called, are available in a variety of sizes, shapes, and colors. Some are designed to fit into a special bra. Others can be attached securely to your chest using a special adhesive. Prostheses range from inexpensive foam inserts to custom-molded replacements with realistic color and texture.

Breast forms are used not just to maintain appearance and sense of balance, but also to relieve the asymmetric strain on posture that may occur after a mastectomy.

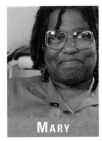

MARY

I went out to get my prosthesis. I went to a very small shop and I took a friend along with me who helped a lot. They have different color prostheses now. I was able to get one that worked for my skin tone. So that was really nice.

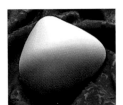 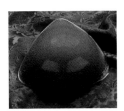 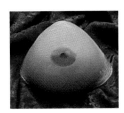

Prostheses are available in light-weight foam, or in natural-weight and -color silicone

QUESTIONS TO ASK YOUR INSURANCE COMPANY:

☐ Does my policy cover the costs of the implant surgery, the implant anesthesia, and other related hospital costs? To what extent?

☐ Does it cover treatments for medical problems that may be caused by the implant or the reconstruction?

☐ Does it cover removal of the implants if this becomes necessary?

☐ If I choose to delay reconstruction and my company changes insurance plans, will I still be covered for breast reconstruction at a later date?

RECONSTRUCTION PROCEDURES

Reconstruction with Synthetic Implants

Synthetic implants are teardrop-shaped pouches that are inserted under the skin to create the form of a breast. In the past, implants were filled with either silicone gel or with saline. Today, silicone-filled implants are available only as part of a research study.

The Question of Silicone

Silicone implants have been used for breast enlargement in over 2 million women over the past 20 years. In the early 90's they were a source of concern because of their possible risk for causing certain collagen diseases, but recent studies have not confirmed these suspicions.

Currently, silicone gel-filled implants are available only to women who are undergoing breast reconstruction, rather than enlargement, and are willing to join a clinical study being conducted by the manufacturer, Mentor H/S, Inc., of Santa Barbara, California.

You'll meet with a plastic surgeon before your mastectomy and choose an implant that will match your other breast and provide a pleasing, symmetrical appearance.

If you're having immediate reconstruction, the plastic surgeon will take over right after the mastectomy, while you're still under anesthesia. This part of the surgery will take about an hour. In order to achieve the most pleasant shape and feel for the reconstructed breast, and to reduce formation of scar tissue around the implant, the implant is often placed under the muscle, rather than directly under the skin.

If the implant is small, the surgeon may be able to insert it without undue stretch to the skin and muscles of your chest wall. If it is too large, a temporary expander will be used for a few months to expand the tissues.

The expander is an elastic bag equipped with a valve. After it is inserted in place, it is filled with a small amount of saline. You'll return to the surgeon's office every week or two to have more saline injected into the expander. Gradually, over three to six months, the skin and muscle will stretch, just like they do over the abdomen during pregnancy. Then the expander will be removed and the permanent implant inserted in its place. A nipple and areola can be created during a future procedure.

The first 24 to 72 hours after your initial implant surgery is when you experience the most discomfort. Your breast will be swollen and tender. Although every woman's recovery time is different, you should be able to resume many of your regular activities after about one week. You will need to wait at least one month before doing anything strenuous.

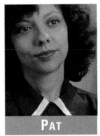

PAT

I had reconstruction at the time of the mastectomy. They put in an expander and slowly filled that for three months and then put in a permanent silicone implant. I am very happy with it.

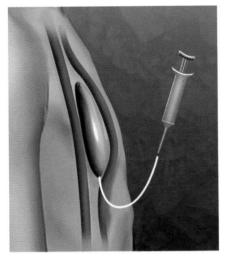

Expander inserted under layer of muscle

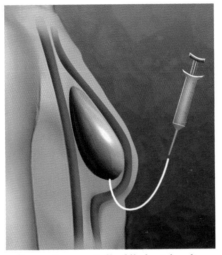

Expander, partially filled with saline

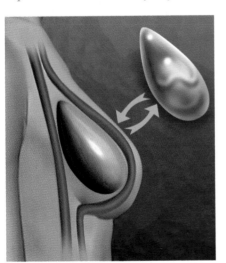

Expander replaced with implant

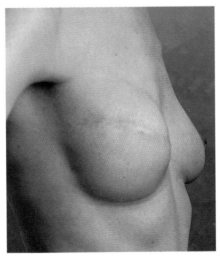

Completed reconstruction

Reconstruction with Your Own Tissues

Breast reconstruction can be done using skin, muscle, and fat taken from another part of your body. This tissue transfer is called a *myo-cutaneous flap*, or simply, a *flap*.

It is a complicated procedure and involves certain risks. Large portions of tissues are moved, and their blood supply is disrupted. There is a possibility that the flap will necrose, or die. This would require removal of the flap, causing significant discomfort and possible deformity.

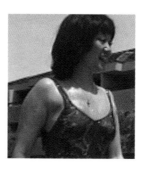

Flaps cause pain both at the donor site and in the breast area. Removal of muscles from their original position can cause pain and weakness, or rarely, a hernia in the donor area.

But, the use of flaps avoids placing foreign materials into your body, and can result in the most natural-looking reconstructions.

There are different types of flaps — TRAM flaps, LAT flaps, and free flaps.

TRAM Flap

The TRAM flap uses one of the rectus abdominis muscles — the "abs," as weight lifters call them. The muscle, fat, and skin are pulled up to the breast area, without cutting the original blood vessels. The flap is then shaped into the form of a breast.

The TRAM flap is the most versatile of the tissue flaps, and can usually create a good match to the other breast for all but the largest-breasted women. No implant is required as is often the case with the latissimus dorsi flap.

The procedure takes three to five hours, and usually requires a four to seven day hospital stay. It also entails an abdominal incision, and does result in

Free Flap

A portion of muscle, fat, and skin are removed from an area such as the abdomen or buttocks and attached to the breast site. Because the original blood supply to the flap is cut, this procedure requires a plastic surgeon who is skilled in micro-surgery — sewing together almost hair-thin blood vessels under a microscope.

The complication rate is the highest with this type of flap, so it is performed only by highly-skilled specialists.

Nipple and Areola Reconstruction

Women who want their reconstructed breast to look as natural as possible may choose to have a nipple and areola reconstruction. This procedure is usually done a few months after the breast reconstruction, so that the breast has had time to "settle" in place.

In one method, a piece of skin is removed from the leg, abdomen, or chest and transferred to the reconstructed breast, where it is shaped into a nipple.

In another method, small flaps of skin on the reconstructed breast are raised and brought together into the shape of a nipple.

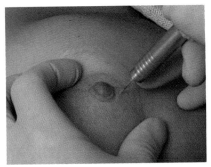

Areola is created by tatooing

The procedures can be done under local anesthesia. Once the skin is healed, an areola is created by tattooing a circular area around the nipple.

WHICH IS RIGHT FOR ME?

Some women are comfortable without reconstruction, viewing their scars as battle scars from a war they waged. Others want reconstruction to erase the visual reminder of cancer, or to enhance their self image. There is no right or wrong answer, and your decision must be respected by those who are close to you, and by your healthcare team.

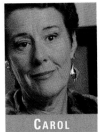

CAROL

One of the really good things about having reconstruction immediately after was that I don't have to be inconvenienced with outside prosthetic devices. I can wear either clothes that are tight or I can wear very low cut clothes, and I don't have to worry about what the impact will be.

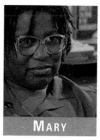

MARY

I considered reconstruction. But I'm not sure if I am going to have it. I have a lot of strong feelings about man-made products in my body and if I can't use the tissues from my own body, I don't think I will ever have it.

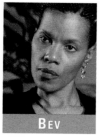

BEV

My surgeon didn't believe in immediate reconstruction. He didn't think the decision should be made at that time. As a matter of fact, he and my plastic surgeon had a disagreement about that, because my plastic surgeon believed that you should do it all together.

Here are some factors to keep in mind when making your decisions:

Synthetic implants:
- They are not lifetime devices, and may rupture or need replacement.
- There are risks of surgery and anesthesia to be considered.
- There are potential risks from implants themselves.
- There is less surgery, less pain, shorter recovery, no additional scar, and less expense than with tissue flaps.

Tissue flaps:
- They are typically soft and normal-appearing.
- There is no artificial implant in the body.
- There is lengthy, extensive, and expensive surgery, with blood transfusions and considerable post-operative discomfort.
- There is an additional scar.
- There is a small but significant risk of the flap "not taking."

Immediate reconstruction:
- You don't have to wake up from mastectomy surgery without a breast.
- One surgery rather than two means lower cost, fewer problems from anesthetic and surgery, and less recovery time.

Delayed reconstruction:
- Provides additional time to make reconstructive choices.
- For the woman undergoing chemotherapy, possibly decreases the chance of infection in the reconstruction area.
- Avoids difficulties in coordinating operative schedules, which may delay surgery.

Radiation Therapy

WHAT IS RADIATION THERAPY?

Radiation therapy is a form of treatment that uses the same type of rays — commonly called x-rays — that are used to create an image of the chest, or of a broken bone. But for treatment purposes, the x-rays are of higher intensity, and deliver much higher doses.

High doses of radiation can destroy the ability of cells to grow and multiply. Both normal and cancer cells are affected, but normal cells have the capacity to recover quickly, while the abnormal, rapidly multiplying cancer cells are

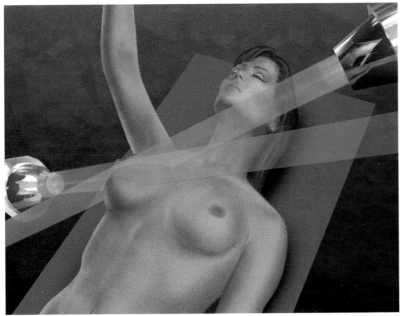

Radiation beams from several angles treat the entire breast area

permanently damaged. Given after a lumpectomy, a course of radiation therapy can help ensure that no cancer cells remain in the breast.

Unlike chemotherapy, which treats the entire body, radiation therapy is considered a *local treatment* because it treats only the site of the original cancer.

Radiation therapy is a painless procedure with few side effects, but it does require daily trips to the hospital for treatment sessions over a period of five to seven weeks.

TREATMENT PLANNING

The goal of radiation therapy is to destroy all cancer cells that may have been left behind in the breast area, while causing as little damage as possible to normal tissues. This requires careful, individualized planning.

Using a *simulation unit* that emits low energy x-rays, a radiation oncologist and his staff will determine the best angles for the high-energy beam to reach the breast area, with as little effect on surrounding tissues as possible. They will then outline the *treatment ports* — places on your body where the beam will be aimed. These ports will be temporarily marked with colored ink. Don't wash these marks off until you're told to do so. Later, they may be replaced by tiny tattoos. These markings will ensure that the radiation beam

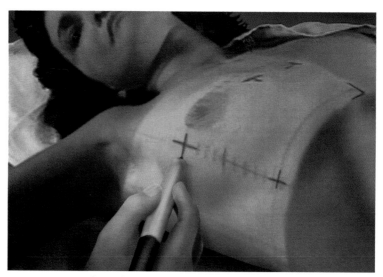

The technologist marks the treatment ports

QUESTIONS TO ASK YOUR DOCTOR:

☐ Why do I need radiation therapy?

☐ How is the radiation oncologist (physician) involved if the treatments are given by the therapists?

☐ How will I evaluate the effectiveness of the treatments?

☐ Can I continue my usual work or exercise schedule?

☐ Can I miss a few treatments?

☐ Can I arrange to be treated elsewhere if I am traveling?

☐ What side effects, if they occur, should I report immediately?

☐ Can I expose the treated area to the sun?

☐ Will I be able to conceive and bear a child after treatments?

is aimed consistently and accurately every treatment session. Some treatment centers prefer to mark the ports with tattoos at the time of simulation.

The simulation session may take several hours. The information obtained will be entered into a computer to develop a treatment plan that is tailored to your particular case.

Sometimes a special cast will be fabricated for your chest to ensure proper positioning, or to avoid skin folds that may interfere with the beam. Special lead blocks may also be custom-made to shape the radiation beam, and protect the normal tissues around your breast.

Once the planning is completed, the treatments can begin.

HOW TREATMENT IS GIVEN

Radiation therapy is administered at medical centers staffed by teams of professionals specializing in radiation oncology. The full course of treatment runs about five to seven weeks, with sessions from Monday through Friday, and rest and recovery periods during weekends. If you have to miss a day or two, discuss the situation with your doctor or nurse. You can make up the days at the end, but the efficiency of the treatment depends on having as few delays as possible.

The first treatment will take longer than the others, in order to make sure the position matches the angles that were worked out during simulation. Since all of this will be a new experience, you may want to bring a friend for moral support.

The treatments are administered by a radiation therapist in accordance with the plan developed for you by the team. Typically, you will arrive at the facility at the appointed time, and will be taken into the treatment room. You may want to bring a Walkman or a book to read in case you have to wait.

Don't use deodorant on the side being treated, because deodorants contain aluminum that may interfere with the radiation beam. You may use a little cornstarch, which can work as a deodorant, or a prescription deodorant recommended by your physician. For the treatment itself, you will wear a

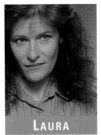

LAURA

The staff would meet me promptly, and take me right in, set me up, and make sure that I was comfortable. So the session went by really quickly, which was great. And they were very kind, very nice people, which made me less nervous. They told me what was going to happen, so I didn't have to worry. It worked out very well.

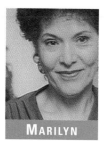

MARILYN

Cosmetically, I had very good results from the treatment. If you look at my breasts right now, you couldn't tell that there was treatment done to one breast as opposed to the other breast. They look exactly the same.

patient gown from the waist up. It may be helpful to wear a two-piece outfit so you can change easily.

You will notice the treatment room has thick concrete walls, and lead-lined doors. This protects those who are not in the treatment area from radiation.

The machine used to administer the radiation is called a *linear accelerator*. The whole set up may seem complex and intimidating at first. But don't be concerned. A TV monitor lets the staff keep you in sight at all times — in case you need anything.

The radiation technologist will adjust the position of the machine according to the previously developed settings, then step out of the room. During the actual exposure you must remain as still as possible. Each exposure lasts only a few minutes and you won't see or feel anything.

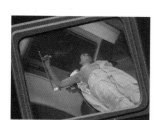

Staff monitors the patient

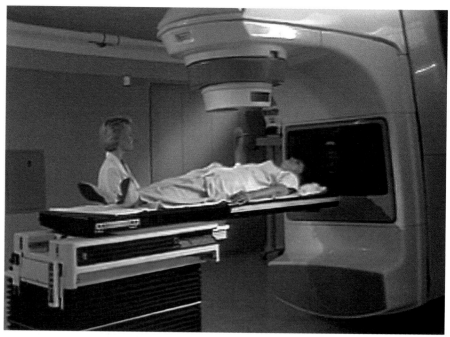

The technologist positions the machine over the breast area

The start of your therapy will depend on whether you are also undergoing chemotherapy. Sometimes the delay may be as long as several weeks or several months. There is little danger of the cancer cells spreading during this delay.

Often you will receive both chemotherapy and radiation treatments. The reason you may need both is because radiation, like surgery, is a *local treatment*, and it is effective against cancer cells in the breast area only. Chemotherapy is a *systemic treatment* — the drugs can reach and destroy cancer cells anywhere in the body. Depending on the practices of the facility where you are being treated, you may have chemotherapy and radiotherapy simultaneously, or be started on chemotherapy, then treated with radiation, then again with chemotherapy.

The Boost

After a full course of radiation therapy you may be given a *boost* — an extra amount of radiation to the area where the tumor was, to ensure that no cancer cells are left untreated. This extra radiation can be given in one of two ways: with an *electron beam*, or by implanting *radioactive seeds*.

The electron beam is the more frequently used method to deliver a radiation boost. The beam contains electrons — tiny particles that can penetrate a short distance into the tissues, and are very effective at destroying cancer cells. You will not be admitted to the hospital for this treatment.

Some therapists prefer to use the *radioactive seed* method to administer the boost. In this case, several pieces of thin plastic tubing, containing tiny pellets of radioactive material will be threaded through your breast, under local anesthesia and mild sedation. You will be admitted to the hospital for three or four days, because the radiation from the seed implants, although very small, may be harmful to some people who may come in close contact with you, such as pregnant women.

SIDE EFFECTS OF RADIATION THERAPY

Radiation therapy is a safe, proven treatment with few unwanted side effects. Most of them are not serious and disappear quickly. The side effects vary from patient to patient, and you may have none or only a few mild ones through your course of treatment. The most common are fatigue and skin

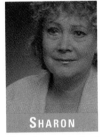

SHARON

The changes in the breast that I noticed is that one's a little firmer. I nursed three babies so the breasts were eh-eh to begin with. I don't notice any other change, except slightly more tan skin.

changes. You will not have nausea or lose your hair, as you might with chemotherapy, and you certainly won't be radioactive.

Most people find that they can go through radiation therapy while maintaining their normal work schedule and lifestyle.

Fatigue

During radiation therapy, the body uses a lot of energy healing itself. Stress related to your illness, daily trips for treatment, and the effects of radiation on normal cells may lead to fatigue. Most people begin to feel tired after a few weeks of radiation therapy. You can help yourself by not trying to do

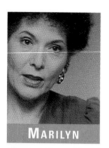

MARILYN

Toward the end of the treatment, I did experience some changes in the breast. I had been forewarned this would happen. There were some skin changes, some coloring changes, some tenderness, and I was given some cream to use. But, I had very little trouble really, compared to what might have happened.

too much. If you feel tired, limit your activities, use your leisure time in a restful way, and try to get more sleep at night.

If you continue working a full-time job while undergoing radiation therapy, talk with your employer about adjusting your work schedule, or try working at home for a period of time.

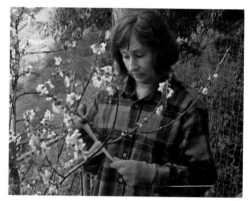

Skin Changes

The energy waves used in radiation therapy have an effect on the skin that resembles the effect of sunlight. Some skin irritation and redness, similar to a sunburn, may develop by the third or fourth week of treatment. Don't rub or scratch the affected area. Use mild soap, being careful not to wash off port markings, if you have any. Wear soft clothing, preferably cotton, and protect the treated area from sunlight. Advise your doctor or nurse at once if your skin cracks or blisters, so that they can instruct you on proper care.

ion Therapy

nt area. Don't use any soaps,
es, cosmetics, talcum powder, or
hout talking with your doctor.

kin. If bandaging is necessary,
outside of the treatment area.
nurse to show you how to apply

, ice pack, etc.) to the treatment
in, so use only lukewarm water

ave the area — but only after
Do not use a pre-shave lotion or

you are undergoing treatment,
ing before going outside. Ask
that contains a sunblock. If so,
product with a protection fac-
een often, even after your skin
Continue to protect your skin
radiation therapy.

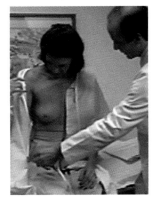

*Skin redness caused by
radiation therapy*

, and tenderness, so you may find
Try using pillows to create a com-
e after treatment.

In addition, you may have tenderness in the breast and chest area for up to a year, but seldom will it be severe enough to require pain medication.

On a long term basis, the breast may become slightly smaller or larger. The breast may also become slightly firmer, but significant hardening is rare.

CHAPTER 7

Chemotherapy

Surgery and radiation therapy are *local treatments* that treat cancer cells in the breast area only. But sometimes a *systemic treatment*, using drugs that can reach all parts of the body, will be added. This treatment can be in the form of *chemotherapy* (drugs that kill cancer cells) or *hormonal therapy* (drugs that prevent cancer cells from growing).

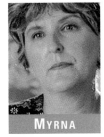

MYRNA

What I associated with chemo was sickness, nausea, not being able to function in my life. The reality has been amazing. I never expected to do as well as I did. I have virtually no problems whatsoever. I've been able to go about my life completely normally.

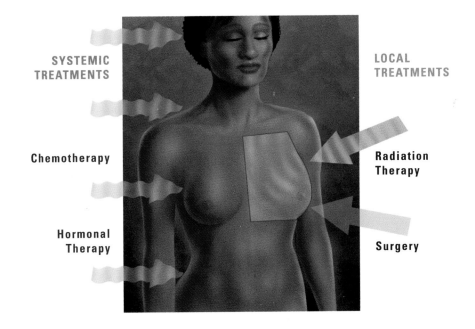

SYSTEMIC TREATMENTS

LOCAL TREATMENTS

Chemotherapy

Radiation Therapy

Hormonal Therapy

Surgery

Why would you need additional therapy if the tumor was already removed with a lumpectomy or mastectomy, and there are no signs of *metastasis*, that is, tumor spread to other areas?

The problem with cancer is that as the tumor grows, cancer cells can break away and travel down blood vessels or lymph ducts to other parts of the body — much the same way as seeds from a weed are carried away by the wind, or float down a river, to grow somewhere else.

In the very early stages, these groups of break-away cells, called *micrometastases*, are very small, and could be destroyed relatively easily. Unfortunately, it is impossible to say whether micrometastases are present, because these very small clumps of cells cannot be found by any method that exists today. On the other hand, if one waits until they grow into tumors large enough to be seen on x-rays or CT scans, successful treatment becomes difficult, if not impossible.

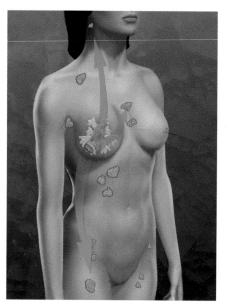

Cancer cells can metastasize to lung, bone, liver, and other organs

So if there is any reason at all to suspect that cells from your tumor have metastasized to other parts of your body before the tumor was surgically removed, you may be treated with chemotherapy or hormonal therapy to destroy those tumor cells as soon as possible.

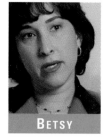

BETSY

I was actually far more fearful and anxious about chemotherapy than I was about losing my breast. And to a large degree that fear and anxiety were unfounded, because the chemo wasn't that bad.

WHAT IS CHEMOTHERAPY?

Chemotherapy uses drugs, called *cytotoxic* (cell-killing) drugs, to destroy cancer cells. It is often used as additional, or *adjuvant* therapy, in conjunction with local treatments like surgery and radiation therapy.

When first told that they have breast cancer, many women panic at the thought of having to go through chemotherapy, because they have heard of it as something that makes you deathly ill, or makes your hair fall out. "Will I have to have chemo?" is one of the first questions that many women ask.

This decision will not be made until after the initial surgery, and after review of all data, including possibly an examination of your lymph nodes for cancer spread.

Chemotherapy is a different experience for different people, and yours may not be as bad as you may be imagining. You may not even have many of the side effects that you have heard or read about. And remember that if your doctor does recommend chemotherapy, you will be enjoying the benefits of one of the most powerful tools for fighting breast cancer.

How Chemotherapy Works

Cells go through several steps in the process of cell division: the DNA in the nucleus forms strands called chromosomes; the chromosomes divide into two sets; the body of the cell enlarges; and finally the cell splits into two identical cells, each with its own set of DNA. Chemotherapy drugs interfere with various parts of this cycle, so that the cells can't divide, or are damaged and can't repair themselves.

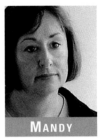

MANDY

I didn't mind going to chemo until the second treatment. I had a severe reaction and became so weak that I couldn't get out of bed. A few days later I awakened with an euphoric feeling. I knew I would be cured. The worst had passed and the rest would be a downhill ride.

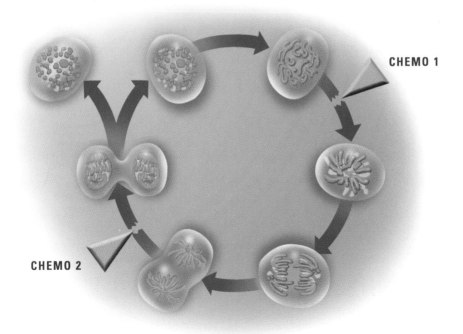

CHEMO 1

CHEMO 2

Different chemotherapy drugs affect different parts of the cell division cycle

Chemotherapy treatment affects both normal cells and cancer cells, but because cancer cells generally divide more rapidly, and are less effective at self-repair, they are more affected by the therapy than normal cells. With proper choice and timing of chemotherapy, tumor cells can be destroyed, without excessive damage to normal tissues.

There are dozens of different chemotherapy drugs, each designed to interfere with a different part of the cell's duplication process. By using a combination of two or three different drugs, it is possible to affect several phases of the duplication cycle and increase the effectiveness of the treatment.

Your oncologist will select the best combination of drugs, based on the characteristics of your tumor, degree of suspected spread, and your general health.

The most common drugs used for breast cancer are cyclophosphamide, methotrexate, 5-fluorouracil (5-FU), and Adriamycin. These are often given in combination: CMF — which stands for cyclophosphamide, methotrexate, and 5-fluorouracil; AC — Adriamycin and cyclophosphamide; or CAF (or FAC) — cyclophosphamide, Adriamycin, and 5-fluorouracil.

Taxol™ (paclitaxel) has been used effectively to treat women with metastatic breast cancer, and is now being evaluated for use as first line therapy.

HOW CHEMOTHERAPY IS GIVEN

Some chemotherapy drugs come in pill form, and you take them just as you would any other pill, but most are given by injection into a vein. These injections can be given in a private doctor's office, in a hospital, or in a cancer center.

Chemotherapy is given in cycles, for example, a dose every three to four weeks. This allows the normal cells in your body to recover between treatments. The full course of therapy takes three to twelve months.

Typical Chemotherapy Day

Your experience with chemotherapy will vary depending on where you receive your treatments, but most healthcare professionals realize that chemotherapy may be a stressful experience for you, and try to make your visit as pleasant as possible.

QUESTIONS TO ASK YOUR DOCTOR:

☐ Do I need chemotherapy? Why?

☐ What drugs do you recommend?

☐ What are the benefits and risks of chemotherapy?

☐ How successful is this treatment for the type of cancer I have?

☐ How will you evaluate the effectiveness of the treatments?

☐ What side effects will I experience?

☐ Can I work while I'm having chemotherapy?

☐ Can I travel between treatments (short business or pleasure trips)?

☐ What other limitations can I expect?

You may make friends with some of the other patients who come for treatment at the same time. Bring a book or a Walkman to listen to music, to make the time go faster. You may choose to practice relaxation or visualization techniques to make the session more pleasant.

Depending on how you feel after treatments, you may want to ask a friend to come with you — for moral support, or to drive you home. If you have problems with nausea, ask your healthcare professional whether you can be pre-medicated with an anti-nausea medication.

Before you receive the scheduled dose of chemotherapy, the nurse will draw your blood. The test results will show whether the treatment has affected the blood-producing cells in the bone marrow, or the function of your liver or other organs. Your blood cell counts typically will be lower. If the results are too far below normal, your oncologist may decide to lower the dose of the medication, or postpone the treatment.

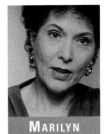

MARILYN

I actually did some modeling during the time I was on chemotherapy, which is sort of a contradiction in terms for many people. But, it really got me through what might have been a difficult period and it made it a very positive year for me.

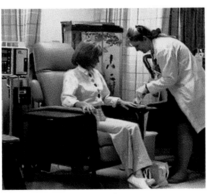

Typical chemotherapy room

If your test results are acceptable, the nurse will take you to the treatment area and start the IV (intravenous line) through which the drug will be injected. If your veins are easy to reach, this will take a few seconds, and feel like a pinprick. Then the drug will be administered. Some drugs are given as a rapid injection, others are dripped in slowly over a longer period — sometimes up to three hours. Generally you won't feel any discomfort.

Sometimes veins are thin, damaged, or covered by a layer of fat, making them difficult to reach. A few IV chemotherapy drugs can be very irritating to the veins, and over the course of treatment, can damage the vein at the injection site. In such cases some women may need a *vascular access device*. These devices, which include *ports* and *PICC lines*, make it easier to administer your medications with the least damage to your veins, and can also be used for drawing blood, thus avoiding needle sticks during clinic visits.

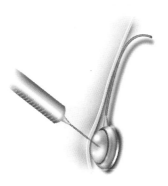

*Chemotherapy drugs
injected through a port*

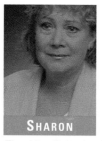

SHARON

*The side effects that I had
with chemotherapy in the
beginning were minimal.
They increased. I gained a
considerable amount of
weight. I don't know if that
was totally the chemo, or that
I was saying, "Ahh, phooey.
I'm going to eat whatever
I want to eat."*

Ports consist of a tube (catheter), attached to a dome-shaped part. The device is surgically implanted under the skin, with the dome placed in the chest or arm, where it will be easily accessible for injections through a needle, but will not interfere with your activities. The catheter is threaded into a large vein near the heart, where rapid blood flow will dilute the drug, and keep it from damaging the lining of the vein.

PICC lines work on a similar principle, but are inserted through the skin of your forearm in the elbow area, rather than surgically under the skin.

Ports and PICCs are removed after chemotherapy is completed.

SIDE EFFECTS OF CHEMOTHERAPY

Anti-cancer drugs work by preventing cells from growing and dividing. The effect is strongest on very rapidly dividing cells, such as cancer cells, but normal tissues can also be affected, particularly the bone marrow, the gastrointestinal or GI tract, the reproductive system, and hair follicles. The side effects will vary with the drug used, and with your own tolerance to it.

While it is important to be prepared for possible side effects of chemotherapy, it is equally important not to assume that you will have all, many, or even a few of them. Many people go through chemotherapy without significant ill effects. If you don't have side effects, it does not mean that the drugs are not working.

Don't compare your treatment with that of another patient, because there are so many different varieties of breast cancer, and so many variables on which the decision is based. Also, do not be alarmed by other women's reports about side effects. Their drugs, and their ability to tolerate them, may be quite different from yours.

It's not likely that you will ever look forward to your chemotherapy days, but a positive attitude, help from your health care team, and support from your friends and family can make chemotherapy a tolerable experience.

The most common side effects are nausea, fatigue, and hair loss.

Nausea

Nausea is a common, and for some women, the worst side effect of chemotherapy. The nausea usually doesn't start until four to six hours after the injection, and may last from a few hours to up to several days, depending on the individual. About one in five women who get CMF, and more of those getting CAF or AC will have nausea and vomiting. In some instances, the nausea can be severe. Sometimes even the fear of nausea itself is so bad that a woman becomes nauseated at the mere sight of the medication, or of the nurse administering it. This is called *anticipatory nausea.*

There are several effective medications available that will control, if not completely eliminate nausea. Discuss this with your healthcare professional, because the right medication may make the difference between completing the full course of therapy or stopping short.

In addition to anti-nausea medications, you may want to experiment with other options such as relaxation or imagery, that have proven to be quite effective for many patients. You can find more information on this subject in Chapter 9.

Nausea can lead to loss of appetite. Since good nutrition is very important to help you fight cancer and retain strength, you should make sure that you have adequate food intake, especially proteins and fluids. Eat small frequent meals avoiding stomach-bloating, carbonated liquids, and increasing the amount of calorie-rich foods.

A few simple steps that can relieve nausea:

- Try breathing through your mouth when you feel nauseated.
- Remove dentures on days you receive drug treatments.
- Avoid fried or other fatty foods.
- Hold a mint or lemon drop in your mouth.
- Avoid eating your favorite foods when you are nauseated, so that you do not develop an aversion to them.
- If the smell of food makes you nauseated, cook outside or take a walk while the food is being prepared.

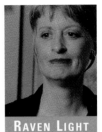

RAVEN LIGHT

I am not a suicidal person. I love life. The first set of chemotherapy that I did was on a Friday afternoon, and that night I vomited all night long. The next day, I just thought of ways to kill myself. I had no libido. I had no interest in sex. I had hardly any energy. It was the pits.

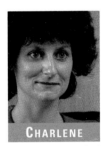

CHARLENE

My physician had given me several different anti-emetics to find the absolute best for me to combat the nausea and vomiting. It definitely was trial and error. Some did not work for me, others helped a lot.

QUESTIONS TO ASK
YOUR DOCTOR:

☐ How can I manage
nausea?

☐ Will I be given medica-
tions to treat side
effects?

☐ Can I take public
transportation home
after treatments?

☐ Should I eat before
I come for my
treatments?

☐ Can I take vitamins or
herbs if I choose?

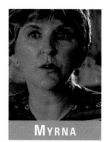

MYRNA

*I had contacted my beauti-
cian and got two wigs before
the hair came out. So the
first day, as soon as it started
falling out, I had the wigs on
and they've been fine.*

Despite the possible loss of appetite, many women notice an increase in weight, rather than weight loss as a results of treatment with most chemotherapy drugs. Weight gain of up to twenty pounds is not uncommon, and can be a distressing side effect for some women.

Fatigue

High doses of chemotherapy can make you feel tired, especially on the first day after each treatment. Adjust your schedule so that you can rest if you want.

Many women find that given some flexibility they can keep a fairly normal level of activity. If you feel totally unable to function at a reasonable level, tell your oncologist about it. Your drug dose may be too high, and may need to be readjusted.

Hair Loss

One of the side effects of chemotherapy that causes women the most sadness is hair loss. If you are receiving the CMF drug combination, your hair may not fall out at all. If you are receiving Adriamycin it probably will. The good news is that hair lost due to chemotherapy always grows back, often thicker and curlier than it was originally.

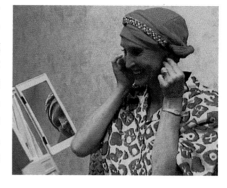

Usually hair falls out gradually, over a period of a few weeks, starting around the third week after beginning chemotherapy. You may find large clumps on your pillow, or in the shower, or notice a lot of hair in your comb. Some women experience a sudden loss of hair.

Consider buying a wig before your hair falls out, and try to pick one that resembles your natural hair. An attractive scarf can be an excellent alternative.

Look Good...Feel Better is a public service program sponsored by the Cosmetic, Toiletry, and Fragrance Association Foundation in partnership with the American Cancer Society and the National Cosmetology

Association. The program helps women manage changes in their appearance resulting from cancer treatment. The program's print and videotape materials are available both to patients and to health professionals.

Call 800-395-LOOK or 800-ACS-2345 or write to them at the address listed in the Resources section.

OTHER SIDE EFFECTS

Some of the less-frequent side effects of chemotherapy can include bone marrow suppression, mouth sores and intestinal problems, and vaginal dryness.

Bone Marrow Suppression

Bone marrow cells, which produce red blood cells, white blood cells, and platelets in your blood, are particularly affected by chemotherapy, and may lose some, or all, of their function, leading to lower blood cell counts.

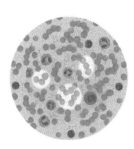

Red blood cells

Red blood cells (RBC's) transport oxygen. The normal value, measured in mgHb (milligrams of *hemoglobin*, the oxygen carrying protein in the cell) is twelve to fourteen. A low red blood cell count, called *anemia*, will generally give you fatigue.

White blood cells (WBC's) help fight infection. A normal WBC count is in the 5,000-10,000 range. There are several different types of white blood cells. The most important for fighting infection are called *neutrophils.*

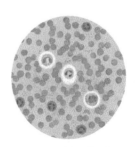

White blood cells

Oncologists use the *absolute neutrophil count* (ANC) to monitor patients under treatment. A neutrophil count of less than 1000 is called *neutropenia*, and makes you susceptible to catching colds or developing various types of infections, including skin wound infections.

Platelets help the blood clot. A low platelet count, below 50,000, can predispose to bleeding. This can take the form of excessive bleeding from wounds, or slow bleeding into the stomach or intestine, which could appear as black stools.

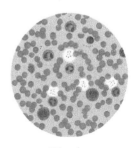

Platelets

Your chemotherapy dose will be adjusted to achieve the maximum effect on the tumor cells, without dangerously impairing the ability of the bone marrow to produce blood cells in sufficient quantities. The health of your bone marrow will be assessed by drawing a blood sample and testing it prior to your scheduled chemo dose.

If your bone marrow becomes excessively suppressed, your doctor may add *colony stimulating factors* to your treatment, to stimulate your bone marrow to produce more blood cells and keep your blood count from getting too far below normal.

Infections

When your white blood cell count is low, your body may not be able to fight off infections, even if you take extra care. Most infections come from bacteria normally found on the skin, in the intestines, and in the genital tract.

Be alert to signs that you might have an infection, such as:

- Fever over 100 degrees Fahrenheit
- Sweating and chills
- Loose bowels
- A burning feeling when you urinate
- A severe cough or sore throat
- Unusual vaginal discharge or itching
- Redness, swelling, or tenderness around a wound, a sore, or an intravenous catheter site.

Report any signs of infection to your doctor right away. This is especially important when your white blood cell count is low. If you have a fever, don't use aspirin, acetaminophen (Tylenol), or any other medicine to bring your temperature down without first checking with your doctor.

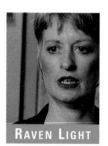

RAVEN LIGHT

One day my roommate came home with the flu, and I caught it. My white blood cell count was so low, I had to go to the hospital.

Preventing Infections:

When your white count is lower than normal, it is very important to try to prevent infections by taking the following steps:

- Wash your hands often during the day. Be sure to wash them extra well before you eat and before and after you use the bathroom.

- Clean your rectal area gently but thoroughly after each bowel movement. Ask your doctor or nurse for advice if the area becomes irritated or if you have hemorrhoids. Check with your doctor before using enemas or suppositories.

- Stay away from people who have diseases you can catch, such as a cold, the flu, measles, or chickenpox. Try to avoid crowds.

- Stay away from children who recently have received immunizations, such as vaccines for polio, measles, mumps and rubella.

- Don't cut or tear the cuticles off your nails.

- Be careful not to cut or nick yourself when using sharp objects.

- Use an electric shaver instead of a razor to prevent breaks or cuts.

- Use a soft toothbrush that won't hurt your gums.

- Don't squeeze or scratch pimples.

- Take a warm (not hot) bath, shower, or sponge bath every day. Pat your skin dry using a light touch. Don't rub.

- Use lotion or oil to soften your skin if it becomes dry and cracked.

- Clean cuts and scrapes right away with an antiseptic.

- Wear protective gloves when gardening or cleaning up after animals and others, especially small children.

- Consult your doctor before receiving any immunization shots.

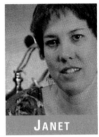

JANET

The first cycle, I didn't really have any side effects. The second one brought cramping and diarrhea, watery eyes, dry mouth, sores in my mouth. With each cycle, the side effects increased. After about three or four, my oncologist cut back the chemicals.

Mouth Sores and Intestinal Problems

The mouth, stomach, and intestines are lined with cells that divide relatively rapidly. Anti-cancer drugs can affect these organs, leading to mouth sores and diarrhea.

It is a good idea to see your dentist before you begin chemotherapy to take care of any preexisting problems such as cavities or abscesses. Ask your dentist to advise you on how to brush and floss during chemotherapy.

Maintaining good mouth care and using a soft toothbrush will help mini-mize sores. If sores do develop, you may find that frozen juices, ice cream, and watermelon can be very soothing.

Oral care during cancer treatment:

If you develop sores in your mouth, be sure to contact your doctor or nurse because you may need medical treatment. If the sores are painful or keep you from eating, you also can try these ideas:

- Eat foods cold or at room temperature. Hot and warm foods can irri-tate a tender mouth and throat.
- Choose soft, soothing foods, such as ice cream, milkshakes, baby food, soft fruits (bananas and apple sauce), mashed potatoes, cooked cereals, soft-boiled or scrambled eggs, macaroni and cheese, custards, and pud-dings. You also can puree cooked foods in the blender to make them smoother and easier to eat.
- Avoid irritating, acidic foods, such as tomatoes, or citrus fruit (orange, grapefruit, and lemon); spicy or salty foods; and rough, coarse, or dry foods such as raw vegetables, granola, and toast.
- Ask your doctor if you should use an artificial saliva product to moisten your mouth.
- Drink plenty of liquids.
- Suck on ice chips, popsicles, or sugarless hard candy. You can also chew sugarless gum.
- Moisten dry foods with butter, margarine, gravy or sauce.
- Dunk crisp, dry foods in mild liquids.

When chemotherapy affects the lining of the intestine, the result may be diarrhea. You can try to eat smaller portions more often, and avoid high fiber foods.

Do not take any over-the-counter medications unless specifically recom-mended by your healthcare provider.

Sexual Side Effects — Physical

Anti-cancer drugs can damage the ovaries, reducing the amount of estrogen in your body, and causing menopause-like symptoms such as hot flashes and vaginal dryness.

Ask your doctor or nurse to recommend a suitable non-estrogen treatment to help reduce hot flashes.

Use a vaginal lubricant if necessary to manage any discomfort during intercourse. To help prevent infection, avoid oil-based lubricants such as petroleum jelly, wear cotton underwear and pantyhose with a ventilated cotton lining, and don't wear tight slacks or shorts.

Chemotherapy, more often than not, damages a woman's ovaries, and may result in infertility, which may or may not be reversible. However, doctors advise women of childbearing age to use birth control throughout their treatment, because some anti-cancer drugs may cause birth defects.

If a woman is pregnant when her cancer is discovered, it may be possible to delay chemotherapy until after the baby is born, or until after the twelfth week of pregnancy, when the fetus is beyond the stage of greatest risk.

Sexual Side Effects — Psychological

Sexual feelings and attitudes vary during chemotherapy. Some women find that they feel closer than ever to their partners and have an increased desire for sexual activity, while others find that their sexual interest declines because of the physical and emotional stresses.

Don't be shy about discussing sexual issues with your nurse or doctor. If you and your partner find it difficult to talk to each other about sex, or cancer, or both, you may want to seek out a counselor who can help you communicate more openly.

QUESTIONS TO ASK YOUR DOCTOR:

☐ Will I continue to have my menstrual periods?

☐ If not, when will they return?

☐ Should I use birth control? What type do you recommend?

☐ Will I be able to conceive and bear a child after treatments?

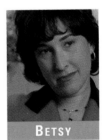

BETSY

What seems to happen a lot of times with chemo, just like with menopause, is that your vagina shrinks and shortens. And you can have problems with dryness. That's the straw that breaks the camel's back sometimes. It's too embarrassing to even think about, let alone talk to anybody.

BONE MARROW TRANSPLANTS

In some cases, breast cancer is discovered at an advanced stage, and is not likely to respond to normal doses of chemotherapy. Very high doses of chemotherapy may be needed. The problem with using higher doses is that they can permanently damage the bone marrow cells. This would inevitably lead to severely low, life-threatening blood cell counts.

In recent years, a procedure known as *stem cell rescue* or *bone marrow transplant* has been introduced. Here is how it works:

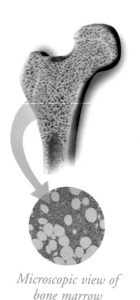

Microscopic view of bone marrow

Before high-dose chemotherapy begins, a sample of bone marrow is obtained by either extraction from a bone in the leg or pelvis, or directly from the blood stream. *Stem cells* (cells which will eventually become blood cell producers) are separated from other cells, and preserved by immediate freezing.

Then one, or several large doses of chemotherapy are administered. These doses are so large that they destroy not only the cancer cells, but also the remaining bone marrow.

After treatment is completed, the bone marrow cells which were removed and saved earlier are thawed and reinjected into the body. This small amount of bone marrow will grow quickly, and begin to produce blood cells.

Generally bone marrow transplants are reserved for high-risk or advanced cancer, where there are at least ten positive lymph nodes, or for recurrent cancer that does not respond to conventional chemotherapy.

Bone marrow transplants are still considered experimental, and many insurance companies refuse to pay for the procedure. The cost can range between $80,000 and $300,000. National and local bone marrow transplant organizations can offer advice on dealing with insurance providers as well as other sources of financial assistance. The National Institute of Health also conducts clinical trials involving bone marrow transplants. Patients accepted into these trials are provided nursing and medical care free of charge.

A number of factors should be considered when making the decision to undergo high dose chemotherapy and bone marrow transplant. On the plus side is the chance of a cure, or the very real possibility of a longer period of disease-free survival. Although extremely unpleasant side effects may be experienced for the first month, a normal lifestyle can usually be resumed after the transplant. On the negative side is the uncertainty that extended survival or cure will be achieved, and the possibility of treatment-related infection, bleeding, organ failure, or, rarely, death.

COMMON CHEMOTHERAPY DRUGS

There are dozens of drugs currently used for breast cancer treatment. Most are used in combinations of two, three, or more. The specific choice depends on the characteristics of your tumor.

Don't be confused because your doctor, nurse and pharmacist may refer to the drugs by different names. *Generic name* is the chemical name of the drug. *Brand name* is the name each manufacturer gives to their specific form of the same chemical. For example, the chemical compound called 5-fluorouracil (its generic name) is marketed as 5-FU by one company, and as Adrucil by another.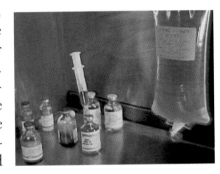

Here is a list of some of the common drugs and their side effects. The description of the side effects is very detailed. Keep in mind that most women do not experience many — or sometimes any — of these side effects.

Adriamycin — *Generic name: doxorubicin*
Common side effects: hair loss, mouth sores, nausea, vomiting, lowered blood counts, damage to the heart muscle, skin damage if drug leaks out of vein during infusion

Report immediately:
- changes in heart rhythm, shortness of breath, or swollen feet. These symptoms may indicate heart damage

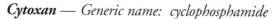

- blood in urine, painful urination, excessive bruising and bleeding, fever or other signs of infection may indicate low blood cell counts

Special Precautions: Drug causes urine to turn reddish in color for a few days, so take special care not to stain clothing. Drink plenty of fluids to insure healthy kidneys and a healthy bladder.

Cytoxan — *Generic name: cyclophosphamide*

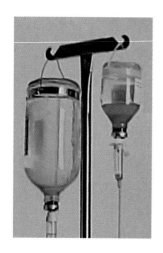

Common side effects: lowered blood counts, nausea, vomiting, loss of appetite, hair loss, loss of menstrual periods, decreased sex drive, bladder irritation, metallic taste in mouth during injection.

Report immediately:

- blood in the urine, painful urination
- fever, chills or other signs of infection

Special precautions: Drink extra fluids so that you can pass more urine in order to keep your kidneys and bladder working well. Try sucking on mints to alleviate metal taste in mouth during injection.

5-FU and Adrucil — *Generic name: 5-fluorouracil*
Common side effects: mild nausea, vomiting, loss of appetite, thinning or loss of hair, skin rash and itching, skin darkening, weakness.

Report immediately:

- fever, chills, sore throat, or other signs of infection
- sores in mouth and on the lips, nausea and severe vomiting
- black, tarry stools; unusual bleeding or bruising
- chest pain, cough, shortness of breath
- difficulty with balance

Special Precautions: Avoid exposure to sun while undergoing treatment.

Methotrexate

Common side effects: Loss of appetite, nausea or vomiting, lowered blood counts, skin sensitivity to sunlight, rash, itching.

Report immediately:

- black, tarry stools; bloody vomit
- diarrhea, sores in the mouth and on the lips, stomach pain
- fever, chills, sore throat or other signs of infection
- unusual bleeding or bruising, blood in urine
- blurred vision, confusion, convulsions or seizures

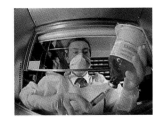

Special Precautions: Drink plenty of fluids. Do not drink any alcohol. Avoid overexposure to the sun. Do not take aspirin or any other preparations containing aspirin or salicylate compounds without first consulting your doctor.

Taxol — Generic name: paclitaxel

Common side effects: allergic reactions such as low blood pressure, shortness of breath, or rash; loss of all scalp, pubic, and facial hair; low blood cell counts; nerve pain.

Report immediately:

- excessive bruising or bleeding
- fever, chills or other signs of infection

Special precautions: Premedication with antihistamines or steroids may reduce allergic reactions during injection. Prepare for long chemo sessions because Taxol is injected over a three-hour period.

CHAPTER 8

Hormonal Therapy

WHAT IS HORMONAL THERAPY?

Chemotherapy uses cytotoxic drugs to kill cancer cells. By contrast, hormonal therapy uses compounds that prevent cancer cells from growing by changing normal body processes.

Hormones are natural chemicals produced by the body to regulate various processes such as blood sugar metabolism, bone growth, or milk production in the breasts. Hormones include such substances as adrenaline, insulin, and estrogen.

Certain types of breast cancers need the female hormones estrogen and progesterone to grow. By using chemicals that block the action of these hormones, it is possible to slow down, or even stop, the growth of cancer cells.

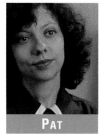

PAT

A low point was when I first started taking the hormonal therapy, because I wasn't sure how my body would react to it, but I've had no side effects, so it's gone well.

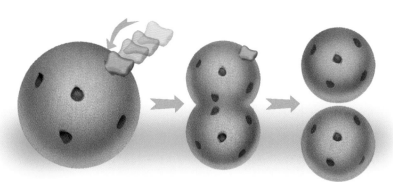

Estrogen fits into receptor sites and stimulates cell division

How exactly is this done? If the cancer is sensitive to estrogen or progesterone, the cells will have certain areas on their surface called *hormone receptor sites.* Hormones fit into these sites like keys into locks, and stimulate the cells to divide.

QUESTIONS TO ASK YOUR DOCTOR:

☐ Did the tests on my tumor show that the cells were sensitive to hormones? (Estrogen Receptor Positive, or Progesterone Receptor Positive)

☐ Should I be treated with hormonal therapy or with chemotherapy, and why?

☐ How will it affect my chance to have children?

☐ How will it affect my sexual function?

Compounds that are similar but not identical to estrogen or progesterone fit into the same receptor sites, and block them, preventing the cell from dividing. Think of it as the wrong key in the lock: it fits, but won't turn, and keeps out the right key.

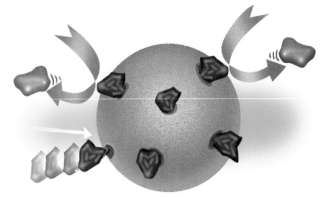

Hormonal agents block estrogen binding sites

Not all types of breast cancer can be treated with hormonal therapy. To determine if hormonal therapy is right for you, a sample of your tumor will be sent to a special lab, where it will be tested for estrogen receptors and progesterone receptors. If the tumor is estrogen receptor positive (ER+) or progesterone receptor positive (PR+), it means that it may be stimulated to grow by one of these hormones.

In this case, your medical oncologist will use a drug such as *tamoxifen,* which binds with the receptors, blocking the effect of natural estrogen, and preventing the cells from growing.

HOW HORMONAL THERAPY IS GIVEN

Hormonal therapy usually starts a few weeks after surgical treatment, and is generally given in the form of a pill taken daily. As with chemotherapy, your hormonal therapy should be supervised by a medical oncologist — a board-certified or board-eligible physician specialist, trained in treating cancer with drugs.

The most common type of hormonal therapy is tamoxifen citrate, or Nolvadex® (its brand name).

A new medication for treatment of advanced breast cancer in women who are postmenopausal is Arimidex®. It works by lowering the body's production of estrogen, and causes few side effects. Another new drug, Zoladex®, was recently approved by the FDA for treatment of advanced breast cancer in pre-menopausal and perimenopausal women.

How Long is the Treatment?
The question of how long to take tamoxifen has been an issue for some time. Clinical studies have shown that there is a clear benefit to women treated for five years, but the benefits beyond that time are uncertain.

Many researchers believe that patients with metastatic cancer should take tamoxifen for as long as the disease is under control.

Who Should be Treated?
Cancer that is confined to the breast area can be treated effectively. Cancer that has spread to areas beyond the breast is much more difficult to treat. Unfortunately, it is not always possible to determine with certainty at the time of diagnosis whether the cancer has spread or not.

Because of this, many clinicians recommend treatment with *adjuvant*, or additional, therapy such as chemotherapy or hormonal therapy, or both, whenever there is a reasonable chance that cancer cells have metastasized to other parts of the body. The reasoning is that while hormonal therapy and chemotherapy may have unpleasant side effects, cancer recurrences are life threatening, and therefore, the benefits outweigh the possible costs.

Younger women, who have not yet gone through menopause, often have estrogen receptor negative tumors, and treatment with hormonal therapy may not be as effective. Post-menopausal women, who often have hormone receptor positive cancers, are more likely to benefit from hormonal therapy.

In general, most clinicians do not use adjuvant hormonal therapy in cases where the tumor is a ductal carcinoma *in situ* — in other words, one that has not spread beyond the confines of the ductal wall.

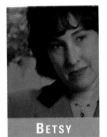

BETSY

In my case, my doctors did not recommend tamoxifen because my hormone receptors were negative. It's actually the one test that's good to hear is positive.

QUESTIONS TO ASK YOUR DOCTOR:

☐ **What side effects should I expect?**

☐ **Can I get pregnant while taking tamoxifen? What birth control method would be most suitable to my lifestyle?**

☐ **What is the latest research data on the safety of tamoxifen?**

☐ **What is the latest research data on how long to take tamoxifen?**

SIDE EFFECTS OF HORMONAL THERAPY

Menopausal Symptoms

Hormonal therapy has far fewer, and less severe, side effects than chemotherapy. Because tamoxifen blocks estrogen, most of them resemble symptoms of going through menopause, such as hot flashes, changes in menstrual periods, and vaginal dryness.

Hormonal therapy also slightly increases the risk of developing uterine cancer, to the same degree as taking estrogen replacement therapy without progesterone for treatment of menopausal symptoms.

Pregnancy

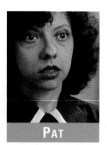

PAT

I would like to have children. Two doctors have said "no," and one has said it's OK. So, we're in limbo right now. If the hormone receptors were negative, there would be no problem with getting pregnant.

Even if tamoxifen stops your periods, you can still get pregnant. Since tamoxifen may be harmful to the fetus, it's important to use birth control if you are sexually active. Use a barrier method, such as a condom or a diaphragm. Do not use an oral contraceptive, or an injection or implant that contains hormones, since they may interfere with your hormonal therapy.

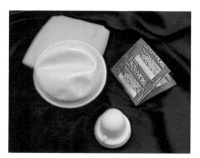

Barrier contraceptives

Secondary Benefits of Tamoxifen

Hormonal therapy with tamoxifen can also have beneficial effects, which you may want to discuss with your oncologist. One of these is the lowering of cholesterol, which may decrease a woman's risk of developing coronary artery disease. This is particularly important for women who are at risk for heart disease, but had to stop their hormone replacement therapy when they developed breast cancer.

Another positive effect is the action of tamoxifen on bones, which may protect women against loss of calcium from bones, and help avoid osteoporosis. Ask your physician if you need to have a simple test called bone densitometry to determine whether your bones are in danger of becoming too brittle.

CHAPTER 9

Complementary Therapies and Alternative Treatments

As you begin to explore your options for treatment, you will undoubtedly hear about things like acupuncture, antioxidants, macrobiotic diets, relaxation and imagery, as well as other *complementary* or *alternative therapies*. While none of these have been proven to cure cancer, some do have definite beneficial effects against pain, nausea, fatigue, or other side effects of treatment.

It's extremely important that you consult your healthcare team before trying any type of complementary therapy to make sure it won't interfere with your treatment.

And remember: complementary techniques are to be used only in conjunction with — not instead of — the treatment recommended by your doctors. That is why most practitioners refer to them as "complementary", rather than "alternative".

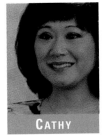

CATHY

Remember spiritually, psychologically, emotionally, that fighting this disease is multi-faceted and treat this disease within you that way. Treat every aspect of it with everything that you've got.

MENTAL TECHNIQUES

Mind/Body Connection

For centuries, people have believed that there is a connection between the state of the mind and the health of the body. How this connection worked, however, was never quite clear.

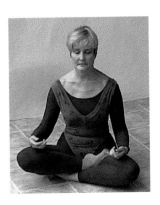

Recently, scientists have identified chemicals, called *neurotransmitters*, by which nerve cells communicate with one another. Neurotransmitters are also involved in the control of emotions. For example, antidepressant medications increase the

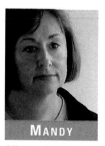

MANDY

I listened to tapes by Bernie Siegel, read motivational literature and practical self-hypnosis books. I took vitamins, especially C, E, and beta carotene. I rode my exercise bike almost daily. When I felt weak , I napped and tried not to feel guilty about sleeping during the day. I believe all these therapies were an important part of my recovery.

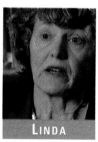

LINDA

I did the Simonton therapy, called "Gettin' Well Again." It had to do with visualizing your immune cells as "warriors." In my case, I visualized them as great white sharks that were attacking any cancer cells that might be remaining in my body. I started feeling a lot better. I had a lot more energy and fourteen years later, I haven't had a recurrence of cancer.

amount of *norepinephrine* and *serotonin* in the spaces between nerve cells. These same neurotransmitters work elsewhere in the body, affecting heart rate and blood pressure, and may even influence the activity of cells in the immune system.

Changes in the state of the nervous system which can occur because of stress or lack of social support, can influence many organ systems. For example, it has been found that people under stress are more likely to develop colds.

Anxiety, grief, stress, and fear of the unknown all seem to have an impact on the body. Learning how to cope with these emotions, using a wide variety of approaches — such as meditation and visualization, spiritual support, and participation in support groups — may help speed your recovery, and benefit your health.

Meditation and Visualization

Meditation has been shown to produce physiological responses such as a decrease in blood pressure, respiration rate, and overall metabolism — all of which contribute to reducing stress on our minds and bodies. Guided imagery or visualization (for example, visualizing natural killer cells gobbling up cancers cells like in the game Pac-Man) is also used with meditation.

While there is no firm proof that meditation and visualization cure cancer, studies have proven that a combination of these techniques can reduce pain and other uncomfortable side effects of cancer treatments.

To demystify the terms "meditation" and "visualization," many physicians simply refer to these techniques as "stress reduction," or "relaxation."

Spiritual Support

Prayer has been one of the most common methods of dealing with illness in all civilizations since prehistoric times. Today, while most would consider prayer to be an unconventional way to treat cancer, many simply accept some form of spiritual support as a basic human need. Prayer, laying on of hands, and many forms of spiritual imagery or inner dialogue have helped patients find the higher strength within themselves to cope with breast cancer and other illness.

Many cancer patients access powerful spiritual experiences directly through their established religious traditions. Even those with negative religious experiences from childhood often find that they are drawn toward a spiritual response by the "spiritual emergency" of cancer. To their surprise, they often find this time the spiritual response is more positive than the religious experiences that disappointed them earlier in life.

Humor / Laughter

Laughter can stimulate endorphins — chemicals that act like opiates in the brain. You might find humor and laughter emotionally healing. In addition, giving yourself time not to think about your cancer can be emotionally beneficial.

While some enjoy standup comedians, others may prefer Marx Brothers movies or sitcom reruns, such as *I Love Lucy*. Writer Norman Cousins discovered that ten minutes of genuine belly laughter had an anesthetic effect that would give him at least two hours of pain-free sleep.

NUTRITIONAL TECHNIQUES

Diet

There's still a great deal of controversy on the subject of nutrition and its effect on breast cancer. So far, there's no scientific data available which proves one diet better than another for breast cancer treatment, although there is some evidence that a low fat diet may decrease the incidence of recurrence of breast cancer in post-menopausal women. Most physicians recommend that patients simply follow established guidelines for good nutrition, with particular emphasis on the need for additional protein and vitamins during chemotherapy treatment. A consultation with a nutritionist will help you learn more about your particular needs.

Macrobiotic diets emphasize whole grains, miso soup, fresh vegetables and beans, with little fruit and no sugar. Special diets such as these may someday prove to be effective for patients with certain types of cancer, but more scientific research is needed in this area.

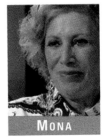

MONA

I immediately started meditation and guided imagery. I went to see a woman, a psychiatrist, who had had a double mastectomy and was very understanding of the problems that I was going through. I felt that I needed to let out a lot of rage and hostility in a controlled environment.

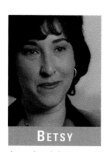

BETSY

I got back into meditation, into bio-feedback, into guided imagery. I cleaned up my diet, took the vitamins that I needed to take, and the herbs, and looked into acupuncture and some other modalities. And I think it really enhanced the way I dealt with chemo. I never threw up. I never lost all of my hair, though I was told that I would.

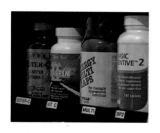

Herbal Therapy

The majority of herbal therapies are based on the belief that they improve organ function. There is increasing evidence from Asian and European countries that some herbs can be effective in fighting cancer.

Since some herbal preparations are extremely potent and may be harmful if used for more than a week or two, practitioners who dispense herbs do so on an individualized basis in accordance with each patient's needs. You should always consult your healthcare professional before beginning herbal therapy, since some preparations may interfere with your treatment.

Vitamins

Physicians recommend vitamin therapy as a complement — not as a replacement — in the treatment of cancer.

Many biological processes in the body lead to the formation of toxic products such as toxic lipid peroxides, which can damage DNA in cells, leading to cancer. Vitamins C, E, and beta-carotene are "anti-oxidant" vitamins commonly used to neutralize these potentially toxic products. In addition, elements such as selenium and copper may be useful, in trace amounts only, to facilitate the defense against toxic peroxides.

It is generally thought by radiation oncologists that antioxidants may interfere with the beneficial effects of radiation, and should be used only with the approval of your radiation oncologist.

Talk with your physician or nutritionist, or contact the NCI or ACS to find out about the latest recommendations on the topic of antioxidants and other vitamins.

OTHER COMPLEMENTARY THERAPIES

Acupuncture and homeopathy are based on the concept that there is a *life force* within our body organs. This life force — an animating factor — maintains the body in a state of health, and predisposes us to disease when it is unbalanced.

Acupuncture

Acupuncture is a technique, first developed in ancient China, which involves insertion and manipulation of needles at specific points in the human body to restore the balance of life force within the body.

The theory behind acupuncture is that there are special *meridian points* on the body which are connected to internal organs. *Vital energy* flows along the meridian lines, and diseases are caused by an imbalance of this flow. Normal flow of vital energy is restored by inserting and twirling needles in the meridian points. Current research studies suggest that acupuncture needles may work by triggering the release of natural pain inhibitors.

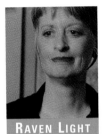

RAVEN LIGHT

For a couple of weeks before my mastectomy, I started doing some Chinese herbs and started seeing an acupuncturist for the first time in my life. So then I continued all through my chemotherapy with my acupuncture and also my "bunch of flower" remedies, which really helped with the terror of going for chemotherapy.

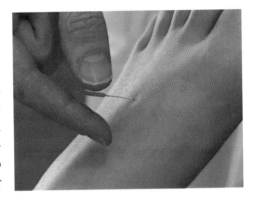

In China, acupuncture has long been used for pain relief, and for treatment of ailments such as arthritis, hypertension, and ulcers. It is now also used as anesthesia during childbirth and some types of surgery. Acupuncture has been used with some success by a number of Western physicians to relieve nausea, pain, or other symptoms associated with cancer.

Homeopathy

Homeopathy was first formulated by German physician Samuel Hahnemann in 1796, and introduced to the U.S. in 1825.

Practitioners of homeopathy believe that minute, highly diluted doses of a medicine offer excellent treatment for the life force, not the physical force, of organs such as the liver, kidneys, or intestines.

Although homeopathy is largely questioned by most American physicians, it is widely used in Europe and Asia.

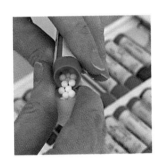

ALTERNATIVE TREATMENTS

Reputable medical practitioners believe that before anything can be safely used as a treatment for cancer, or any other condition, it must undergo rigorous testing and evaluation, using large numbers of patients, and objective analysis of the results.

But from time to time, a new product suddenly appears, and is promoted as the new alternative to standard medical treatment for cancer. Most of the time, the claims are founded on a few poorly documented cases of alleged "cures," and sometimes on nothing but a promoter's greed or ignorance.

An example is *laetril* — a substance made from apricot pits, that was presented as a cure for cancer, based on the claim that cyanide contained in the apricot pits killed cancer cells. Scientific studies, and personal experiences of patients who tried the treatment on their own, have proven laetril to be useless or even harmful, and there have been reports of deaths from cyanide poisoning.

One of the most recent non-approved products being promoted is *shark cartilage*. However, an FDA-approved clinical trial of a shark cartilage preparation called Benefin failed to prove its effectiveness in fighting breast cancer.

How to Approach Alternative Therapies

Obtain Objective Information: Become an informed health consumer. Speak with people who have gone through the treatment. Ask about the advantages and disadvantages, risks, side effects, costs, and results they experienced.

Consult your Healthcare Provider: Discuss all treatments with your physician or primary healthcare provider, who needs to have a complete picture of your treatment plan.

Examine the Provider's Expertise: Inquire about the training and expertise of the person administering the treatment (for example, their certification or license to practice in their particular field).

Consider the Costs: Many alternative treatments may not be reimbursable by health insurance.

CHAPTER 10

Clinical Trials

Rather than relying on standard approaches to cancer management, scientists are constantly searching for better ways of dealing with the disease. Many women diagnosed with breast cancer may benefit from this research by participating in *clinical trials*.

WHAT ARE TRIALS?

A clinical trial is an evaluation of a new way of managing cancer. Some trials are designed to see if a new drug will be effective in treating or preventing cancer. Other trials evaluate new ways to diagnose the disease.

Clinical trials help improve the quality of care, now and in the future. One such trial conducted a number of years ago showed that lumpectomy with radiation treatment was as effective as the established practice of removal of the entire breast. As a result of this trial, many women today can enjoy the benefits of breast-conserving surgery.

Clinical trials are not random attempts at finding some new way of dealing with cancer.

New treatments are first tested in laboratories, using animals. If there is evidence that the treatment may be effective, it is evaluated further with actual human cases, usually with advanced stages of the disease.

To reach the clinical trial stage, where large numbers of patients are used, the treatment method or drug must show good evidence of potential benefit, at an acceptable risk level.

QUESTIONS TO ASK ABOUT A CLINICAL TRIAL:

☐ What is involved in terms of tests, treatments, and additional time commitments?

☐ What results can be reasonably expected in my particular case?

☐ What are the currently accepted treatments and how do they compare to the trial?

☐ What would my financial commitment be and how can I cope with it?

☐ Will I need to be available for follow-up testing indefinitely?

If the clinical trial confirms the benefits, the drug or treatment will be made available to all patients.

HOW ARE TRIALS CONDUCTED?

Every trial is conducted according to a *protocol* — a set of guidelines that spells out exactly what will be done and when. Large numbers of patients are selected according to very specific criteria — age, stage of cancer, previous treatment, and so forth.

The patients who meet these criteria are divided into groups. Most trials consist of a *control group* (patients who are receiving standard therapy) and a *treatment group* (those who receive the new therapy that is being evaluated). The treatment group always receives treatment that is considered to be at least as good, and possibly better, than the standard treatment. Sometimes the control group receives a *placebo* — an injection or a pill that looks like the drug being evaluated, but has no medicinal value.

Patients are assigned to one of the two groups by a random, computerized system, where neither the patient nor the physician has control over the selection process. In addition, neither the patient nor the investigator knows which group the patient was placed in, until the end of the trial. This process is called *double-blind* randomization, and helps avoid bias on the part of the patient or the treating physician.

A central agency keeps all the records of the selection, and can reveal them if the need arises. Sometimes, if one group is showing a significantly better response than the other, the trial is terminated, and all patients are given the better treatment.

IS A TRIAL RIGHT FOR ME?

If you are thinking about participating in a trial, ask your healthcare professional how to proceed. Generally, you or your physician can obtain information about ongoing trials from the National Cancer Institute's hotline called PDQ, or from the local chapter of the American Cancer Society.

You and your physician will review the lists of requirements for various trials to see whether or not you might qualify for one of them. If you do, be

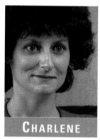

CHARLENE

When the word "research" was first presented to me, I felt very fearful: Is this something that's only been tried on me? Am I the research rat? But when I learned more, I realized that it wasn't like that. I felt very fortunate knowing that I was getting aggressive therapy and that I would only benefit from it.

sure to find out what is involved in terms of tests, treatments, additional time commitments, and side effects, and evaluate whether or not you can live with these terms for an extended time.

After a thorough explanation, you will be asked to sign an *informed consent form*, to show that you understand the issues involved, the expected benefits, the possible side effects, your rights and responsibilities, and the possible outcome.

You will be asked to follow the schedule of treatments and tests as closely as possible, in order to make the information obtained scientifically sound. However, your participation is completely optional and voluntary. You can leave the trial at any time. If you drop out, you will not be penalized in any way, and you will still be entitled to the best standard treatment available.

Patients in both the control group and the treatment group benefit from participating in the trial, because trial protocols usually call for more frequent tests, more frequent visits to the hospital, and more thorough examinations, which generally translates into a higher standard of care.

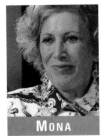

MONA

When I was asked to be on a research study, it was very carefully explained to me by my doctor and his nurse. I took a copy of the papers home, and as a matter of fact, sent one to a female physician friend of mine. We talked on the phone about it. I felt that I would be carefully watched and carefully monitored. So I had no hesitation.

RECENT DEVELOPMENTS

Two promising approaches to breast cancer prevention have been reported recently.

In mid-1998, a large trial showed that tamoxifen reduced the risk of developing breast cancer by 45%. The results were so clear, in fact, that the trial was stopped two years before the scheduled date, and women in the control group who were receiving a placebo were offered tamoxifen.

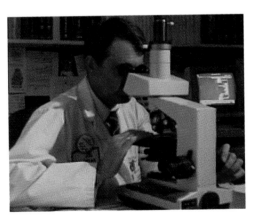

Another development is the discovery that tumors that produce high levels of an oncogene called HER-2/neu may be more resistant to hormonal and chemotherapy. Treatment with an antibody drug called herceptin can delay the growth of the tumor.

Researchers continue to find new uses for a drug called Taxol (paclitaxel), developed from the yew tree. One trial showed that Taxol could be effective in treating early as well as advanced cases of breast cancer.

CHAPTER 11

Life After Cancer

You had your last dose of chemotherapy, or your last radiation treatment. The surgical scars are beginning to heal. As your energy and confidence return, you'll be able to explore the many options for moving forward from the cancer experience to a new life.

MENTAL RECOVERY

Healing the Mind

A diagnosis of cancer is a threat to your self-esteem, body image, sexuality — even to your survival. You must realize that life will never be the same after such an experience, and that your consciousness will have been changed forever by it. Take time to grieve the loss. This grieving process is an important first step toward the healing of the mind.

Going through the cancer experience is likely to cause bouts of confusion, sadness, and despair. These are normal reactions, and will come and go, and gradually decrease as you adjust to your diagnosis. But there are specific times during the course of treatment and recovery when these bouts are more likely to occur.

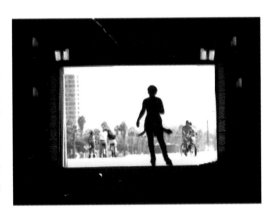

QUESTIONS TO ASK YOUR DOCTOR OR NURSE:

☐ What can I do if I wake up at night worrying about my cancer?

☐ Will the cancer cells that may have spread to other parts of my body start to grow when I stop taking chemotherapy?

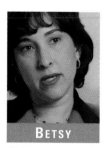

BETSY

At least while I was in chemotherapy, I was actually doing something to take charge of the cancer, to kill any cancer cells that might be running amuck in my body. When I walked out of the chemo suite for the last time, there was a feeling of, "Now what? Where do I go from here?"

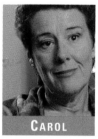

CAROL

I found it really important to learn to laugh at myself. The whole thing is a disaster, and if you can find some little bits of humor in it, you might feel better. Remember, the universe is proceeding exactly the way it's supposed to be, whatever happens to you. So you just put one foot in front of the other and do the things that need to be done.

Most women experience their highest level of anxiety when they come home from the hospital after surgery, because coming home means leaving most of the medical team behind and resuming normal activities.

Another time women may feel anxious or depressed is when their chemotherapy or radiation treatments end. There may be a feeling of panic at the thought that you are not being treated any more. This post-treatment anxiety is quite natural, and will gradually diminish as you regain confidence.

Some women notice that they are particularly anxious on the anniversary dates of their diagnosis or surgery. These are the so-called *anniversary reactions*. In addition, many women also may have *check up anxiety* just before their scheduled follow-up visit to the physician.

Depression

Episodes of anxiety and depression are to be expected. What is important is to distinguish between what you can cope with on your own, what can be supported by family and friends, and what requires professional help.

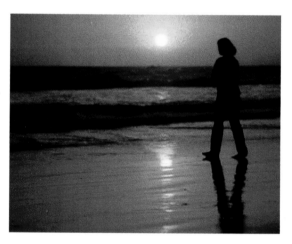

"Feeling blue" means that you can still enjoy parts of life. It is a natural response called reactive depression. This level of depression is normal, and most women can cope with it with the support from family, friends, or support groups.

You may want to plan fun activities such as going out with friends or seeing a movie around the times when you normally feel depressed or blue. Another approach is to try to get out of your mind and into your body, so to speak. Physical activity stimulates the body to produce certain chemicals called endorphins that help restore a sense of well being. Exercise and sports are valuable tools for helping you manage anxiety and depression.

Other effective techniques include relaxation and visualization, described in the chapter on Complementary Therapies.

If you haven't already, consider joining a support group. You should have no trouble finding one that matches your lifestyle and your particular needs. You will find a list of resources for referral to support groups at the end of the book.

Clinical Depression

There are forms of depression that are unlikely to improve on their own. Some of the feelings that signal that you may have a *clinical depression* requiring treatment include continuous feelings of sadness, feelings of worthlessness or guilt, excessive fear of the future, and lack of interest in intimacy or sex. If you have some of these feelings, tell your physician about them.

If you have thoughts about suicide, call your physician or nurse immediately.

Clinical depression can be treated. It may involve counseling, medications, and perhaps physical exercise and stress reduction techniques. Your physician will be able to refer you to the appropriate specialist.

And remember, you should never feel embarrassed to seek professional help. It is not a sign of weakness — no more so than going to a surgeon for a lumpectomy.

PHYSICAL RECOVERY

Regular Follow Up

Even after the most complete treatment, there's always a chance that cancer will recur in the breast, in the lymph nodes, or in distant parts of your body. Most recurrences happen two or three years after surgery. The longer you go without a recurrence, the greater are your chances of remaining free of disease. But you can never say that the cancer has been completely cured.

Because of this possibility, you need regular follow up visits with a healthcare professional. It could be your family physician, your oncologist, or your breast surgeon. Usually you'll be seen as often as every few weeks immediately after treatment, and perhaps only every six months later on. There is

QUESTIONS TO ASK YOUR DOCTOR OR NURSE:

☐ What can I do about feeling excessively tired?

☐ Why have I lost interest in intimate relations with my partner?

☐ Why can't I sleep or relax or feel interested in anything?

☐ Why can't I stop feeling that I am going to die because of the cancer?

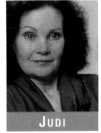

JUDI

A few months ago, my son and I went for a trip to the Grand Canyon, and that's something I've always wanted to do. I felt much, much better than if I had just stayed at home feeling sorry for myself. And I find that if my attitude is positive I do feel much better than if I allow myself to become depressed.

no "right" schedule. What's important is to have a single person in charge of the follow-up care.

What does follow up involve? Most physicians suggest a physical examination every six months, to look for signs of local recurrence — new lumps within the breast after lumpectomy, or tiny hard nodules in the surgical scar after mastectomy.

In addition, mammography will be scheduled on a regular basis, and you may have a number of blood tests that will assess the function of your liver, bone marrow, and other organs. A chest x-ray also may be done. Other tests, such as CEA (a protein found in the blood of patients with cancer) and bone scans, are not used routinely, but are appropriate in certain situations.

BSE

One of the components of follow-up is your monthly breast self-examination. A proper BSE should include looking at your breasts in various positions in front of a mirror, as well as feeling the entire breast area with your fingers. The best way to learn how to do BSE, if you don't already know, is to ask your healthcare provider to teach you, or to acquire a copy of a good breast self exam video, such as *The New BSE with Marriette Hartley*. More information on this program is available in the Library section at the end of the book.

How to Do BSE

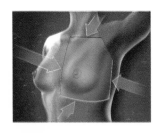

Using a mirror, check the shape and size of your breasts, and the color and texture of your skin, first with your arms down, then with your arms in the air. Try to learn what's normal for you, so that you can spot any changes immediately.

Check your breasts in two other positions — pushing down on the hips, to tighten your chest muscles, and bending forward at the waist, with your arms relaxed. This will help you spot dimpling — the tugging on the skin or nipple often caused by a growing tumor.

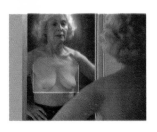

Next, lie down with a folded towel under your shoulder. Extend the arm out at an angle to spread the breast tissue more evenly. You will need to examine the breast as well as the area where breast tissue may be found — from the armpit, to the breast bone, and from the collar bone to the bra line.

Use three middle fingers to examine the breast. Use the pads because they're more sensitive than the tips. Keeping the fingers straight with the pads flat against the breast, make three dime-sized circles. One just lightly, one deeper, one deeper still. This will enable you to check the full thickness of your breast.

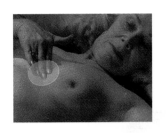

When you move your hand, don't lift the fingers away from the skin, to avoid missing a spot. Cover the entire area, spot by spot, going up and down in strips about as wide as your three fingers.

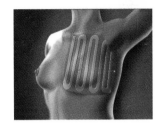

When you've finished, lower your arm and examine your armpit for possible lymph node enlargement. Then check the other breast the same way.

Ask your nurse or your doctor to show you how to examine a mastectomy scar. Irregular lumpiness is common after a lumpectomy, but local recurrences may feel like tiny firm beads along the incision line.

If you had a mastectomy, you should have mammograms of the other breast.

Mammography

Every woman who has had breast cancer should have a mammogram once a year, regardless of age.

If you had a lumpectomy, the films may be more difficult to interpret, so make sure that previous mammograms are available for comparison.

Care of the Arm

After breast surgery, and particularly after a lymph node dissection, your arm on the side of the surgery may feel numb and tingly or you may have shooting pains due to nerve regrowth.

You may also have decreased range of motion in the shoulder as a result of nerve damage.

Your healthcare professional will tell you which exercises are appropriate to help your arm regain its mobility and strength. It is very important to follow the exercise schedule faithfully so you can recover your full range of motion. You will find a description of some of the exercises in the mastectomy section of the Surgery Chapter.

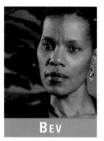

BEV

I never really understood it, but I've had so many... you know, offers... after my mastectomy, I almost think I should have had this a long time ago. It could be men are attracted to my drive to live, because I was faced with an illness that could have caused my death.

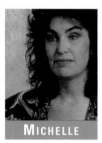

MICHELLE

It has been approximately two years since my reconstruction. I feel very much like a woman. And I don't just feel normal, I feel very attractive. I feel like I have my sexuality back and I feel that I would be attractive to any man.

Lymphedema

As you have read in Chapter 4, lymphedema is swelling of the arm due to scarring of the lymph ducts after surgery or radiation. This condition occurs in approximately ten to twenty women out of a hundred, sometimes months or years after surgery. It may severely affect the strength, mobility, and appearance of the arm.

It is important that you always follow your medical team's recommendations about how to avoid injury to the arm to reduce the chances of developing lymphedema. Regular exercise, maintaining a normal weight, and gentle massage can help prevent this condition.

If your arm becomes red, swollen, or feels hot, call your doctor at once. Keep the arm elevated above your head and periodically pump your fist until you can have it examined.

The National Lymphedema Network (800-541-3259) is an excellent source of information. You will find a detailed description of their services in the Resources section.

INTIMACY AND SEXUALITY

Your Self Image

We live in a society that considers breasts to be an important aspect of a woman's attractiveness. The loss of a breast after a mastectomy, or even a slight change in shape after a lumpectomy may have a serious impact on a woman's confidence. "Will I be attractive?" "Will I still be loved?" are valid questions that need to be answered in a woman's mind.

Doubts about your appearance and attractiveness are normal, but you should not let them affect your self-image. Remember, there is much more to sexuality and pleasure — and to you as a person — than the shape or presence of a breast.

The critical issue is not the loss of the breast itself, but the way you and your partner treat the loss. Open communication is very important. Many couples find to their surprise that the patient is more concerned about the loss of her breast than her partner is.

Resuming Sexual Activity

Some women and many of their partners worry about when and how it is acceptable to resume sexual activity after breast surgery. Sometimes the partner may avoid physical contact simply out of fear of causing discomfort to the woman.

There is nothing about breast surgery itself that would require a delay. Even if you still have a dressing, or drains and stitches, there is no reason not to engage in intimate contact. The decision is based more on your emotional state than on your physical readiness.

Often it will have to be you who first mentions your fears or needs, because your partner may feel that these issues are too personal. Do so as early as possible. The more time passes without open discussion, the harder it becomes to deal with the subject.

If you're not ready, make it clear to your partner that not wanting to make love is not an act of rejection, and that you may welcome other forms of physical intimacy.

Some women who have had a mastectomy purchase sexy lingerie, or have intimacy in subdued lighting to help take the edge off the presence of a surgical scar, without reducing the feeling of closeness and excitement.

If you have loss of sensation in the breast or nipple area, you may need to gently guide your partner, indicating what is now pleasurable to you.

Hugging, touching, holding, and cuddling may become more important, while sexual intercourse may become less important. Remember that what was true before your cancer remains true now: there is no one "right" way to express your sexuality. It's up to you and your partner to determine together what is pleasurable and satisfying to both of you.

The American Cancer Society has a free booklet on sexuality that may be helpful. Contact your local unit or the national office for copies.

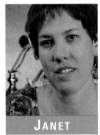

JANET

It didn't affect my sexual relationship at all. It maybe enlightened it because I think that our love grew from the experience. It definitely didn't get worse.

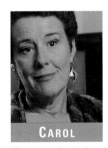

CAROL

The sexual relationships that I was in after the mastectomy required communication that hadn't been there before. I had to be able to tell people what would feel good.

Side Effects of Treatment

If you did not yet go through menopause, chemotherapy or hormonal therapy may stop your periods temporarily or permanently. If you are young, your periods are more likely to return than if you are approaching menopause.

Even if you have no evidence of menstrual bleeding, you may still be ovulating — and therefore may get pregnant. Be sure to discuss birth control with your physician. Do not take oral contraceptives, which contain the female hormones estrogen and progesterone, without talking with your oncologist. Effects of these hormones may stimulate growth of certain cancers, as well as interfere with hormonal therapy.

The anti-estrogen drug tamoxifen used in hormonal therapy may actually increase ovulation, making effective contraception particularly important.

Breast cancer does not rule out the possibility of having children, and many women choose to do so. If you're in your child-bearing years and would like to have a baby, it is very important to discuss this issue with all the physicians on your team, including your oncologist, radiation therapist, pathologist, and surgeon. It is important that they review all the details of your case — such as cancer type, degree of spread, amount of radiation you received, and so on — before advising you on whether it is safe for you to get pregnant.

NEW BEGINNINGS

New Perspective

The breast cancer experience can be a powerful incentive to reorder priorities and see life from a different angle. To make a point of finding something enjoyable in every day, in every task. A reminder to stop and smell the roses.

Breast cancer can also be a liberating experience. You may decide to do something you always wanted to do — write poetry, travel, or spend more time with your children.

This may be a good time to adopt healthy habits, such as good nutrition, increased physical activity, and other lifestyle changes.

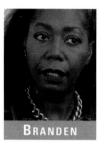

BRANDEN

I started a journal before the mastectomy, when I was first diagnosed with breast cancer. Later, I got a grant from the National Endowment for the Arts, the journal turned into a play, and premiered it at the Los Angeles Theater Center.

Good Nutrition

Good nutrition may speed your healing after surgery and help you during chemotherapy. Later on, balanced diet, with proper amounts of protein, fats, carbohydrates, and vitamins will help you feel younger and stay healthier. Currently, there is no evidence that breast cancer can be prevented by a low fat or any other type of diet, although certain diets may affect the incidence of other cancers, such as colon cancer.

Physical activity

You may have done arm exercises as part of your post-surgical recovery. Physical activity will strengthen and energize you, so don't neglect the rest of your body. A regular exercise program will help you stay stronger and feel younger. There is also evidence that moderate physical exercise can improve the work of the immune system.

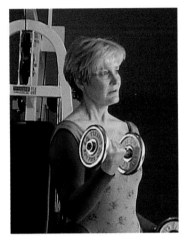

Lifestyle Changes

As a breast cancer survivor you may be at an increased risk for other types of cancer, such as ovarian cancer, lung cancer, or skin cancer. This may be an excellent reason to stop smoking and to take better protective measures when you expose your skin to the sun.

Other lifestyle changes, such as relaxation or meditation, may help you in your personal and professional life.

Recommendations for Your Family Members

Although the majority of cases of breast cancer are not hereditary, having a first degree relative with breast cancer increases the likelihood of developing the disease. A good word of advice is to inform your family members of your diagnosis, and suggest that your daughters or sisters be particularly aggressive in practicing early detection. The current recommendations include yearly mammograms starting either at age forty, or at an age that is ten years younger than yours at the time of your diagnosis, whichever is earlier.

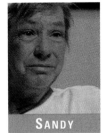

SANDY

You know, when something like this happens, then you realize what you've been missing. It's a great feeling, to walk out in the morning and smell the clean air. I never did that before.

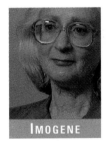

IMOGENE

I can't state too loudly to women with breast cancer that in order to have a fuller and richer life you need to use the rage that you have creatively. If you have some talent, use it. And do something with it. Get your rage out. I think that's the most important thing for survival, and for a fuller, richer life.

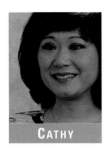

CATHY

One of the most wonderful things about my life after breast cancer is that I've spent a lot of time helping other people. I think breast cancer is a remarkable disease because so many women who are survivors come through that experience and say, "I want to do something to help other people through this."

Getting Involved

As you regain your physical and emotional strength, consider the needs of your fellow breast cancer survivors who may be in earlier, or in more difficult stages of their recovery, and could benefit greatly from someone guiding them through the experience.

The American Cancer Society's Reach to Recovery Program, Y-ME, WIN Against Breast Cancer, the Susan G. Komen Foundation, and other organizations listed in the Resources section need volunteers who can help other women in their struggle with breast cancer.

One simple way you can get involved in the fight against breast cancer is to buy the breast cancer postage stamp. The stamp was approved by Congress in July of 1997. It costs a few cents more than a regular stamp. The extra proceeds will go toward breast cancer research. By using the stamp, you not only provide financial support, but you also raise awareness of the cause. To order your stamps, call 1-800-STAMP 24.

CHAPTER 12

A Guide for Your Partner

As the partner of a woman with breast cancer, you're probably in as much pain and turmoil as she is. The coming days and months will be challenging. You'll have to deal with your own feelings, as well as give the woman you love the support she needs. A positive attitude will help both of you get through the ordeal.

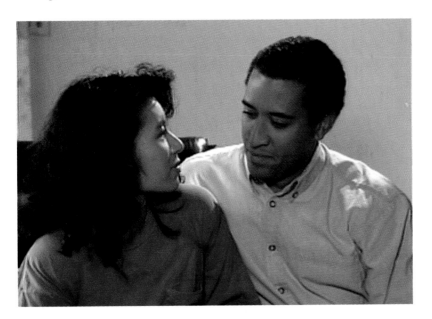

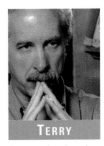

TERRY

I remember hearing a lot from doctors that there wasn't an awful lot you can do, other than hope. I think this is the time when you need to set a direction in terms of your attitude, and building the strength to say, "I'm going to fight this and learn to do what I have to do."

WHAT IS BREAST CANCER?

You may know breast cancer as something that requires a big operation and leaves the woman disfigured, or something that is treated with chemotherapy, causing hair to fall out. And something that women usually die of.

In reality, breast cancer that is diagnosed early is one of the most treatable forms of cancer. There has been enormous progress in breast cancer management in the past twenty years. There are effective combinations of treatments that can kill cancer cells, and surgical techniques that give cosmetically pleasing results.

In the next days or weeks, you should review the appropriate chapters of this book with your partner, and learn with her. Understanding breast cancer and its treatment will help you regain a feeling of control over your life.

UNDERSTANDING YOUR FEELINGS

"The doctor told me I have breast cancer." These may be the most painful words you'll ever hear from someone you love. Words that bring out a flood of emotions — shock, disbelief, confusion — and the inevitable question, "Is she going to die?"

Dealing with these issues is a lot to handle. On top of this, you have an even bigger task. You have to quickly come to grips with your own emotions, so that you can become the main source of support for the woman you love. In the coming days and weeks, you may be called upon for a variety of reasons — to take notes during medical visits, drive her to chemotherapy sessions, listen without judging, or hold her close when she needs it.

You may feel overcome by the feeling that somehow you must make it all better, and be frustrated when you find out you can't. There is no easy answer, and no shortcut. Accept what you are feeling. Don't be embarrassed. You are facing a serious problem, and it is normal to feel scared, confused, and weak.

Breast cancer can stress all aspects of your relationship. There may be a disruption of lifestyle, as treatment schedules or treatment-related financial burdens prevent you and your loved one from participating in the activities you are used to. The roles each of you played in the relationship may change, and you may find that you are now responsible for tasks you are unaccustomed or unwilling to tackle. You may have to deal with the side effects of her treatment, such as fatigue, nausea, vomiting, or loss of sexual

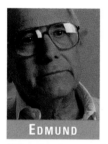

EDMUND

When the doctors told us that Joan had cancer, my first thought was "Is she able to survive this emotionally?" And it did not ever enter my mind that I was going to lose Joan, because we knew that she was positive in her thinking and I was positive in my thinking. And all it was is just a bug that had to be removed.

drive. And there will be the turmoil of having to make important decisions while facing the uncertainties of the future.

Fear, anxiety, and sadness will affect how the two of you communicate. Acknowledge these feelings. You can be strong and supportive without holding everything inside. In fact, sharing your feelings honestly with her is the best thing you can do. Rather than losing confidence, women with cancer appreciate the fact that their loved ones can express emotion in such a trying situation. This sharing improves communication and strengthens your relationship.

If you find it too hard to express these feelings to your partner, you can find a support person for yourself. A friend, another family member, a religious leader, or a counselor can help you verbalize what you are feeling, sort it all out, and work on a plan of action.

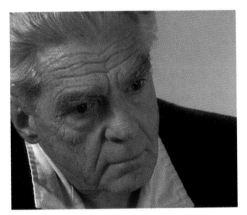

During the first weeks after her diagnosis you will probably feel like you are riding an emotional roller coaster. There will be days when after a conversation with your loved one, or a visit to the physician, everything will seem under control, and you will feel strong and optimistic. But at night, negative thoughts will begin to creep into your head, and you'll feel like all is lost, and there is no hope. You may spend the night pacing, or crying, or wondering what you'll do if you lose the woman you love. By morning you'll remember that there are excellent treatment options, and that her outlook for a healthy life is much better than it seemed a few hours ago.

These swings of feelings are painful and exhausting, but they are normal. The good news is that with time these emotional tidal waves get smaller and smaller — until they are just ripples in a pool, and you find that you can deal with them.

QUESTIONS TO ASK HER DOCTOR:

☐ Do you have any pamphlets, videos, or CD-ROMS about breast cancer we can take home and review?

☐ Is there a Resource Center or patient library in the facility where you practice?

☐ Who would you recommend we see for a second opinion?

☐ Can you put us in touch with women who you treated for breast cancer, and with their partners?

WHAT DO I DO NOW?

You are in a position to contribute greatly to the peace of mind and success of treatment for your loved one. What you do and say in the first few minutes and days after she hears her diagnosis will make a great difference in how she feels about it herself, and will play an important role in her physical and mental recovery. Try to be as positive and supportive as you can.

One of the most constructive actions you can take is to get involved in her care. Learn all you can about the disease and the most current treatment options. Accompany her on visits to her healthcare specialists. Your presence will provide emotional support and a second set of ears.

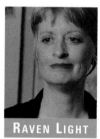

RAVEN LIGHT

I'm a highly sexual woman and so is my lover. And I know that in the past she has made comments about not wanting to be lovers with handicapped women. Once I was diagnosed, I kind of expected that she would just go her way, but she didn't at all. She stayed with me the whole time. From her I learned unconditional love for the first time in my life.

Bring a list of questions you want answered. Take notes, or use a tape recorder so you can review the information you received. It may take time to feel confident about how much you understand. Breast cancer treatment is a complex topic, and no one can be expected to grasp all the details on the first pass.

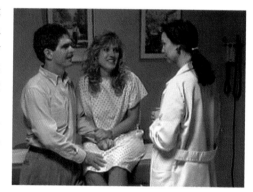

If you or your partner feel you need a second opinion, don't hesitate to ask her physician for a referral, or seek one on your own. For something as important as breast cancer treatment, you owe it to yourselves to leave no avenue unexplored, and no reputable healthcare professional will resent your request.

Bear in mind that the diagnosis of breast cancer is almost never an emergency. You and your partner have several weeks to make important treatment decisions. Don't let anyone or anything rush you.

Above all, remember that the final decisions about treatment will be your partner's. Being supportive and helpful does not mean taking over completely.

What She Needs From You

Emotional Support

Along with the fear of losing her femininity, and possibly her life, what a woman fears most at this time is that the one she loves will abandon her.

Emotional support is perhaps the single most important factor you can contribute. Knowing that you will be there for her, no matter what, and that you still find her lovable, desirable, and attractive will help her face her diagnosis and tolerate her treatments better than anything else.

You can also help by creating a safe place for her to express her emotions. This means allowing her to grieve in her own way, without making judgments about the "appropriateness" of her behavior.

If you find verbal communication to be difficult, and choose to hide in your job or in an outside activity, she may perceive this behavior as a withdrawal of your love. Her well-being, and the survival of your relationship itself, depends on your willingness to communicate openly. You don't need to make long speeches. Holding her hand, sitting close to her, putting an arm around her, will communicate how much she means to you in ways words can't express.

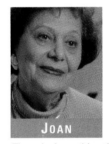

JOAN

There isn't anything that we didn't share. Every word, every feeling, every little thing that went on, we shared. I don't think I could have gone through it without him. He has never said anything that hasn't been, "You're beautiful." And he wasn't afraid to look at the scar and say, "Oh, look how much improvement, isn't that great?" He made me feel wonderful. He made me feel like a star.

A few simple techniques that will improve communications

- Make opening statements that let your partner know you're willing to listen. Comments like, "how do you feel about..." let her know it's okay to open up on an emotional level.

- Reassure her that she has been truly understood by repeating what you heard in your own words.

- Use nonverbal (body language) techniques to convey how you feel about her. Hand-holding, and looking at her when she speaks tell her that your love and concern are real.

- Avoid judgmental comments like, "you shouldn't..." or, "don't say that." Such statements block true communication by minimizing or invalidating the other person's feelings.

- Be careful with comments like, "don't worry," or, "nothing will happen." Having a positive attitude doesn't mean being unrealistic.

SIGNS THAT MAY INDICATE CLINICAL DEPRESSION

- Ongoing sadness and negative statements ("I'm not worth anything anymore." "I hate my life.") lasting a period of weeks rather than days.

- Withdrawing from all normal activities or social/family interactions.

- Physical complaints: sleeplessness or sleeping too much, continual tiredness, over- or under-eating.

If your partner displays any of these patterns consistently for two weeks, notify her doctor.

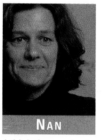

NAN

I think the mastectomy scar was easier to look at than looking at the biopsy scar. The breast was bruised and it looked very damaged. So the mastectomy scar, even though it was much more traumatic, was very clean. To me, it wasn't terribly shocking, and there was a sense of relief in it.

Most people, especially men, are upset by tearful outbursts, so your first reaction to her crying may be an attempt to "fix it" or somehow "make it all better." But remember that tears are a healthy response. You and she know that there is no easy fix, and to pretend otherwise only delays the grieving that must take place before healing begins.

Anger is also a normal response. Breast cancer is no one's fault, but anger needs an outlet. She may lash out at the closest person during such times. The important thing to remember is that despite what she says, she is not angry at you, but at her loss of control over her life. This stage will pass, and she needs to know you'll still be there for her. Help direct that anger into action, to fight against the cancer and depression.

Some women withdraw and refuse to share their feelings, rejecting your efforts at being close. This may be the most difficult reaction to deal with, and may require outside help to reestablish open communications.

Some degree of depression is also to be expected. How do you know if your partner's mood is normal, or if she has severe depression? This is an important question, because depression can adversely affect her treatment. It is normal to have short periods of sadness, "blue moods," apathy, or loss of interest in daily activities. You can help her overcome these feelings on your own. But a more serious form of depression, called clinical depression, with prolonged feelings of sadness and loss of interest in all activities, should be managed by a professional.

Once chemotherapy or radiation treatment is completed, your partner may be overcome with feelings of panic or powerlessness that come from the perception that she is no longer actively fighting the disease. It is important to acknowledge these feelings, then focus on the positive aspects of completing the treatment.

There is scientific evidence that a positive mind-set can lead to an improved outcome. A supportive and upbeat attitude on your part will be contagious and is one of the best ways to help her through the weeks or months of treatment.

Reassurance About Her Appearance

An unreconstructed mastectomy, or complete loss of hair caused by chemotherapy will result in dramatic changes in appearance that will often make the woman feel that her partner will no longer find her attractive. A woman's acceptance of her changed body often depends on her partner's reaction to it. You need to prepare yourself accordingly. Your reaction to these changes will have a great impact on how well she tolerates them.

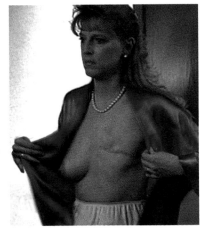

Looking at the mastectomy scar or reconstructed breast for the first time can be very frightening. Bear in mind that once it is healed, the scar will look infinitely better. The swelling, bruising, stitches, and bandages will be replaced by a clean white line. Try to be as sensitive and accepting as you can. Give her the type of response that you'd like to hear if you were in a similar situation.

Some women have no trouble looking at the surgical site together with their partners at the earliest opportunity. Others choose to view the scar gradually, sometimes alone, or in subdued lighting, or under the cover of an attractive nightgown. Respect her wishes, and be positive and reassuring when you look at her. What is important is not how her chest looks, but the fact that she is still the same woman you love.

Sexual Intimacy

When is the right time for resuming sexual relations? There is nothing about breast cancer that would prevent intimate contact, even if the dressings and drains are still in place. The deciding factor is your partner's, and your, readiness.

Surgery can be exhausting and debilitating. Tenderness around the surgical site, or loss of sensation in the nipple can interfere with physical pleasure. Wearing a natural-looking prosthesis, or having her partner touch other areas of her body, can help a woman refocus sensation and regain interest in intimacy.

QUESTIONS TO ASK HER DOCTOR:

☐ Will there be loss of sensation in the breast area?

☐ Will chemotherapy cause her hair to fall out?

☐ Can we see pictures of what the surgical scar could look like?

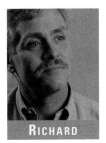

RICHARD

I was intrigued by the fact that Carol had one breast that was quite different than the other. But as far as being shocked or like, don't touch or anything like that, no. That part did not bother me. It was just, "Ok, this is Carol. This is part of the package. I like the package."

Chemotherapy can cause nausea and weakness that can leave minimal energy for sexual relations. There is usually a period of time just before the next treatment, in which your partner will have had time to recover and may find physical contact more pleasurable.

Preoccupation with the cancer and its treatment will probably decrease your and her interest in sexual intimacy. There are a number of small things you can do to rekindle her sexual interest. Make a date with her, give her a foot rub, take a shower together, watch an erotic movie. Try new positions that may be more comfortable.

Help with Daily Activities
After she comes home from the hospital, your partner will have days of physical and emotional exhaustion, and will need your help to handle even the most mundane daily activities. Some women need more help than others. The hard part may be determining how much help she wants. Ask her what she feels like doing on a given day. Look for physical signs of how tired she might be, but avoid "babying" her. Too much help may be as inappropriate as too little.

SUGGESTIONS FOR FRIENDS WHO WANT TO HELP

- Stop by and bring a newspaper

- Bring the mail or other materials from the office

- Help redecorate a room

- Organize a getaway weekend for both of you

- Drop by and watch a favorite TV program

- Drive her to a chemotherapy session

- Invite the whole family out for a meal

Her doctor will provide instructions for her care after the surgery, but be sure to ask for clarification if you have questions. The goal is to return to as normal a life as possible without causing either of you excess stress.

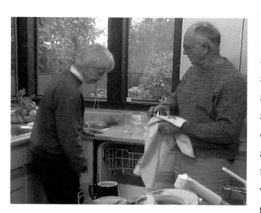

In the early stages of her treatment she may be overcome with a barrage of well-wishing friends and relatives. You will need to act as the gate keeper — or appoint a specific person to channel the good will. A good approach is to delegate specific tasks to various people, such as walking the dog, shopping for groceries, driving the car pool, keeping other friends informed, and so on. That way, everyone feels involved, and the necessities of life are attended to.

If you have children at home, they will need the time and support your partner may not always be able to give them. One of the most helpful things you can provide is a special time or activity that all family members can participate in — for example, renting a movie or going on a picnic.

You also may be required to deal with financial or insurance issues. There are some things you can do to make an unpleasant task much easier:

- Contact your insurance company at the time of diagnosis to find out their policies on hospital admissions, additional medical opinions, and filing of claims and billing.
- Keep a written record of your contacts with insurance company representatives, including names, dates, and times.
- Write down appointment dates and doctors' names. Get a copy of all billing forms for procedures, medications, and supplies used.
- Keep all bills, charges, and related forms together in one place for easy retrieval later.
- Don't forget to keep up insurance premiums. You'll be glad you remembered this critical step later.

MEETING YOUR OWN NEEDS

Finding Support for You

The combination of emotional stress, your regular work, and added activities around the home can take a toll on you. You can't afford to exhaust yourself physically or emotionally. Seek assistance from family or friends whenever you need. A simple request may be all they are waiting for to pitch in.

When your feelings threaten to overpower you, confiding in close friends or family can help ease the emotional burden you carry. Talking to other partners of women with breast cancer can also give you concrete ideas on how to cope.

You should also consider joining a support group. Groups for partners of women with breast cancer are often assembled according to age, professional background, or other criteria.

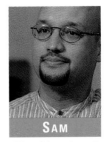

SAM

When I found out that Terry had cancer, I had no family up here and my friends only had pity for me, and that was the last thing I really needed. I needed to find a place where I could sit and talk and share my fears that I was going to lose my wife. That's where joining a support group really helped.

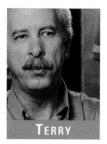

TERRY

It's hard to go and talk to the guys at the office about your wife's mastectomy. I mean, guys just don't open up that much and so there were things that I didn't have anybody to really talk to about. It would have been helpful to have had some support element, whatever it might be.

Do not be embarassed by the prospect of joining a group. It is not a sign of weakness. The group will give you an opportunity to discuss the feelings and fears that you may be reluctant to share with the woman you love.

Your partners' healthcare provider can help you find a support group in your area that matches your needs and lifestyle.

Dealing with the Workload

As the primary support person, you will have a major role in keeping up with your family's daily activities during a difficult time. There will be times when you may feel overwhelmed by the entire burden. Before that occurs, sit down with your partner and make plans:

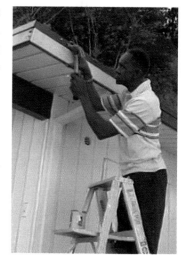

- Make a list of tasks that need to be done on a daily basis (food preparation, child care). Try to concentrate on activities that really are essential, and put off the unnecessary niceties.

- As people contact you and ask "How can I help?" give them specific tasks that will be truly helpful for you and your partner.

- If you have the financial means, you may want to hire help. Even having someone a few hours a week can ease the situation.

- If you have children, get them more involved in the daily activities.

My Experience as the Partner of a Woman with Breast Cancer

Ten years ago, at the age of 43, my wife went for what we thought would be a routine mammogram of a lump I found in her breast five days earlier. Just as I was starting to realize that she had been gone too long, the radiologist called. "Dr. Lange, we are looking at your wife's mammograms. It looks like she has a malignancy." Just like that. The message was particularly devastating because there wasn't that moment of confusion, that buffer of uncertainty about what I just heard, to soften the blow. I knew what "malignant" meant... as in cancer, mastectomy, chemotherapy, death. I stopped thinking, got in my car, and went down to the radiology facility to pick my wife up.

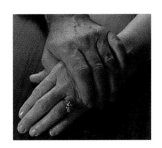

The most important contribution — sometimes I think it was the only contribution — I made to my wife's recovery, was the attitude I took toward her illness. The thought of being left alone to raise two young children without the woman I loved was too frightening a prospect. So I simply decided she was not going to die, and that was that. It was not an option. It was not acceptable. It was my will against mother nature, and I was determined to win the battle. In retrospect, we both feel that somehow that mind-set, however irrational, made the difference.

Another perhaps equally significant form of support was my wholehearted, unequivocal, and immediate assurance to her that I absolutely did not care what form of surgery she may need, and would love her and find her attractive no matter how she looked. Even today, ten years later, she says that it was this attitude that helped her retain her self-image.

In terms of logistical support, "relative wrangling" was definitely a challenge. Relatives tend to have an exaggerated (often grossly exaggerated) response to a diagnosis of cancer. "Oh, my God, how terrible, the poor thing... (read: "she's going to die"). What are you going to do?" To avoid the negative feelings such outbursts would generate, I decided to paint a much rosier picture of her prognosis, and insisted that no one treat her as a sick person. With this attitude adjustment, our families became valuable sources of support throughout Mandy's treatment.

Resources

On the following pages you'll find an extensive list of groups, organizations, and businesses that can help you in your fight against breast cancer. They are divided into categories of general resources, sources of help with appearance, and professional organizations.

GENERAL RESOURCES

The American Cancer Society
National Office:
1599 Clifton Road NE
Atlanta, GA 30329
404-320-3333 or 800-ACS-2345
Website: www.cancer.org

The American Cancer Society (ACS) is the nationwide community-based volunteer health organization dedicated to eliminating cancer as a major health problem by preventing cancer, saving lives from cancer, and diminishing suffering from cancer through research, education, and service.

Free booklets, videos, and other materials are available from your local chapter or by calling 800-ACS-2345.

ACS also operates the *Reach to Recovery* program which can match you with a volunteer who has had the same kind of treatment you are considering. *The Look Good... Feel Better* program helps women deal with changes in their appearance caused by cancer treatment.

The Australian Cancer Society
70 William Street
East Sydney NSW 2010, Australia
02 9380 9022
Website: www.cancer.org.au

An Australian organization similar to the American Cancer Society.

Australian New Zealand Breast Cancer Clinical Trials Group
Department of Clinical Oncology
Newcastle Mater Hospital
Waratah NSW 2298, Australia
+61 2 4921 1155

A group dedicated to the research of breast cancer in Australia and New Zealand. Contact them for more information on the latest clinical trials being conducted.

Breast Cancer Care
Kiln House, 210 New Kings Road
London SW6 4NZ
0500 245 345 (United Kingdom)

Breast Cancer Care is an organization in the United Kingdom that offers free information, help and support to those affected by breast cancer. Their services include a volunteer service, national help-line, prosthesis fitting and a wide range of information from booklets to audio tapes.

Black Healthnet
Home Page: www.blackhealthnet.com

An internet resource for health issues affecting the African American community.

Breast Cancer Early Detection Program /
Breast & Cervical Cancer Control Program
California Department of Health Services
P.O. Box 942732, MS-294
Sacramento, CA 94234-7320
800-511-2300

The California Department of Health Services and the
Center for Disease Control and Prevention fund programs which provide free clinical breast examinations
and mammograms to low income, uninsured, or under-
insured women. The emphasis is on women over 50
but some services are available for women 40-49. The
California program also covers diagnostics.

Women in California can call the toll free number to
find out if they qualify and to get referrals to participating providers in their area. For programs outside
of California, contact your state health department
and ask for the Breast and Cervical Cancer Program.

California Breast Cancer Organizations
8775 Aero Drive #302
San Diego, CA 92123
619-569-9283

A coalition of breast cancer organizations throughout
California, educating, empowering and advocating for
California women.

Canadian Breast Cancer Network
1000, 170 Laurier Ave.
10 Alcorn Avenue, #200
Toronto, Ontario K2P 2N2, Canada
613-788-3311

A Canadian network of groups and individuals with the
goal of helping people affected by cancer.

Canadian Cancer Society
National Office:
10 Alcorn Avenue, #200
Toronto, Ontario K2P 2N2, Canada
613-788-3311

A national community-based organization of volunteers, whose mission is the eradication of cancer and
the enhancement of the quality of life of people living
with cancer.

Cancer Care Inc.
1180 Avenue of the Americas, 2nd Floor
New York, NY 10036
212-221-3300: For a Cancer Care social worker.
800-813-4673: Toll-free counseling line.
Website: www.cancercare.org
E-Mail: info@cancercare.org

A social service agency that helps patients and their
families cope with the impact of cancer. Services
include professional counseling, financial assistance,
information and referral, education programs, and
insurance counseling, at no cost to the client. Direct
services are limited to the greater New York metropoli-
tan area, but callers will be referred to similar assistance
available in their areas.

CancerBACUP
3 Bath Place, Rivington Street
London EC2A 3JR, United Kingdom
Information: 0171 613 2121 or 0800 181 199
Counseling: 0171 696 9000 or 0141 553 1553(Scotland)
Website: www.cancerbacup.org.uk

CancerBACUP is a leading national charity in the U.K.
providing information, counseling and support for people with cancer, their families and friends. It is staffed
by specialist cancer nurses and professional counselors.
CancerBACUP publishes booklets on specific cancers,
treatments and on living with cancer.

Gilda's Club
195 West Houston Street
New York, NY 10014-4872
212-647-9700

A free cancer support community for people living with cancer, their families and friends. Provides social and emotional support through support groups, lectures, workshops and social events.

Institute for Health and Healing Library
2040 Webster Street
San Francisco, CA 94115
415-923-3680 (recorded information) or
415-923-3681 (direct line)

Medical library for the general public. The collection includes current information from professional medical literature, popular health publications, and alternative therapy resources. Books and tapes are available for sale through the bookstore catalog.

Kids Konnected
P.O. Box 603
Trabuco Canyon, CA 92678
Hotline: 714-380-4334 or 800-899-2866 (CA only)
Website: www.kidskonnected.org
E-mail: JWH@kidskonnected.org

Kids Konnected provides friendship, understanding, education, and support to kids who have a parent with cancer. Kids Konnected offers support groups in three age ranges from 3-17. All groups are run by kids and led by Ph.D. child psychologists. A telephone hotline, monthly newsletters, camps, workshops, and social events are some of the many services.

Mautner Project for Lesbians with Cancer
1707 L Street, NW, Suite 500
Washington, DC 20036
202-332-5536
Website: www.mautnerproject.org

Provides support services to lesbians with cancer and their families. Educates lesbians about cancer, and healthcare professionals about working with lesbians.

National Alliance of Breast Cancer Organizations (NABCO)
9 East 37th Street, 10th Floor
New York, NY 10016
800-80-NABCO
Website: www.nabco.org.
E-mail: nabcoinfo@aol.com

The National Alliance of Breast Cancer Organizations is a leading non-profit resource for information about breast cancer, and represents a network of more than 350 organizations. It offers a wealth of up-to-date, accurate information on all aspects of cancer..

The Breast Cancer Resource List published annually by NABCO is considered one of the best guides for finding organizations that can provide information, support, and education; lists of publications and videos, including resources available in Spanish; and personal resources, such as places to find wigs, prostheses, and other items.

National Breast Cancer Coalition (NBCC)
1707 L Street, NW, Suite 500
Washington, DC 20036
800-NBCC-838
Fax: 202-265-6854
Website: www.natlbcc.org

Advocacy and action to eliminate breast cancer.

National Cancer Institute
Cancer Information Service
Office of Cancer Communications
Bethesda, MD 20892
800-4-CANCER (1-800-422-6237)
Hawaii, on Oahu: 808-586-5853
Alaska: 800-638-6070
Website: cancernet.nci.nih.gov

The National Cancer Institute (NCI) is part of the
National Institutes of Health and is the federal government's principal agency for cancer research and
control.

The Cancer Information Service (CIS) of the NCI
offers free written materials and information about
cancer prevention and control, treatment, support services, medical facilities, second opinion centers, and
clinical trials. The hotline is operated by a network
of authorized comprehensive cancer centers. Spanish
speaking staff members are available. All services are
free.

CancerFax, a service of the NCI, provides treatment
information summaries from the Physician Data Query
(PDQ) for health care professionals and patients; information on supportive care, screening, prevention, and
anticancer drugs; as well as fact sheets, news, and bul-
letins from the NCI. Spanish versions are available.
CancerFax can be reached at 800-624-2511.

National Lymphedema Network
2211 Post Street, Suite 404
San Francisco, CA 94115
800-541-3259 or 415-921-1306
Website: www.lymphnet.org
E-mail: nln@lymphnet.org

A non-profit organization that provides assistance and
information to women with lymphedema.

National Women's Health Network
514 10th Street NW, Suite 400
Washington, DC 20004
202-347-1140

A public-interest organization devoted only to women
and health. Advocacy for legislative issues.

NHMRC National Breast Cancer Centre
153 Dowling Street
Wooloomooloo NSW 2011, Australia
02 49 334 1700

This center operated by the National Health and
Medical Research Council provides information and
resources for women in Australia.

Oncolink
Home Page: oncolink.upenn.edu

An internet-based resource, designed by the University
of Pennsylvania Medical Center, to collect and dissemi-
nate information relevant to the field of oncology to
patients, families, and healthcare providers.

Quebec Breast Cancer
Information Exchange Network
Centre hospitalier de l'Université de Montréal,
Hôtel-Dieu Campus
3840 Saint-Urbain Street
Montréal, Quebec H2W 1T8, Canada

An organization providing information, support and
resources for French speaking women in Canada.

Salick Health Care, Inc.
8201 Beverly Boulevard
Los Angeles, CA 90048-4520
213-966-3400
Fax: 213-966-3680
Website: www.salick.com

Salick is a provider of diagnosis and treatment for patients with illnesses requiring sophisticated, long-term care, in the areas of cancer, kidney failure, organ transplantation, and certain immunodeficiency diseases. Services are provided at outpatient facilities (hospital-based and freestanding), selected inpatient sites, and the patient's home.

Salick presently operates eleven Comprehensive Cancer Centers and eight diagnostic and treatment Breast Centers. Through its INFUSX subsidiary, Salick provides infusion, nutritional, and related services in patients' homes.

SHARE

1501 Broadway, Suite 1720
New York, NY 10036
Hotlines: 212-382-2111 or 212-719-4454 (Spanish)
Office: 212-719-0364

A non-profit, self-help organization that provides support services for women with breast or ovarian cancer, and for their families and friends. It offers peer counseling, support groups, hotlines in both English and Spanish, educational and wellness programs, and advocacy opportunities. All services are free of charge. SHARE also heads SHARE-A-WALK, an annual public awareness and fundraising event.

Sisters Network, Inc.

8787 Woodway Drive, Suite 4207
Houston, TX 77063
713-781-0255

An African American breast cancer survivor support group which offers emotional and psychological support as well as medical research, education, and awareness programs, and a national newsletter.

The Susan G. Komen Breast Cancer Foundation

5005 LBJ Freeway, Suite 370
Dallas, TX 75244
800-I'M-AWARE (800-462-9273)
Website: www.breastcancerinfo.com

The mission of the Susan G. Komen Breast Cancer Foundation is to eradicate breast cancer as a life-threatening disease by advocating research, education, screening, and treatment. Komen is the nation's largest private funder of research dedicated solely to breast cancer. Volunteers work through chapter and Race for the Cure® events across the country, funding education and screening projects in local communities for the medically underserved.

The Women's Cancer Resource Center

3023 Shattuck Avenue
Berkeley, CA 94705
510-5489272

Founded by Jackie Winnow, who died of breast cancer, the center provides information on breast cancer and health-related issues for women, referrals, educational forums and workshops. Several support groups meet regularly and a full library is available in a comfortable environment. The center has become a model for grassroots cancer activism across the nation and is well known throughout the lesbian community.

Women's Information Network Against Breast Cancer (WIN ABC)®

19325 E. Navilla Place
Covina, CA 91723-3244
626-332-2255 or 619-488-6300

WIN ABC is a national non-profit organization that provides rapid access to up-to-date information, education, and support to breast cancer patients and their families.

The Breast Aid Program® disseminates information free of charge in the form of pamphlets, books, video and audio tapes, a WIN Resource Guide, mammography screening and breast self exam information, and referrals, as well as information and referral to other support organizations, programs, and patient advocacy groups. Trained information specialists provide telephone support on a case by case basis.

The Breast Buddy® Program trains breast cancer survivors to educate and support newly diagnosed patients. The Breast Buddy® Program for Indigent and Underserved is currently under development for national replication.

Y-ME National Breast Cancer Organization
212 W. Van Buren Street, Fourth Floor
Chicago, IL 60607
Hotline: 800-221-2141 or 800-986-9505 (Spanish)
Website: www.y-me.org
E-mail: help@y-me.org

Chicago-based Y-ME has eighteen chapters in the United States and Canada. The organization provides a national hotline staffed by breast cancer survivors, as well as referrals for medical care and information on finding or starting support groups. Y-ME also maintains a wig and prosthesis bank for women who cannot afford them.

The Y-ME Men's Hotline (800-221-2141) offers support to patients' partners.

The YWCA Encore Program
624 9th Street, N.W., 3rd Floor
Washington, DC 20001
800-95-EPLUS (800-953-7587)
Home Page: www.plasticsurgery.org

A program run by local YWCAs to provide supportive discussion and rehabilitative exercises for women who have been treated for breast cancer.

APPEARANCE

Belle-Amie, Inc.
800-700-2807 or 714-756-9512

A provider of customized breast prostheses. A Belle-Amie representative will make casts of your torso before and after your mastectomy. These casts will then be used to create a life-like breast form that matches the weight, texture, and skin tone of your natural breast.

Bio-Portraits, Inc.
3176 Pullman, Suite 118
Costa Mesa, CA 92626
714-662-7675

This company produces custom breast prostheses made of breathable, skin-like materials designed to capture the subleties of each woman's breast, including the slope, shape, color and texture.

Friends Boutique
at the Gillette Center for Women's Cancers
Dana Farber Cancer Institute
44 Binney Street, Ninth Floor
Boston, MA 02115
617-632-2211

Adults and children with cancer can find a wide variety of specialized products and services in one location. Personal care products, support services and educational materials are tailored to meet the cancer patient's needs.

Nearly Me
800-877-3626

A line of premium-quality breast prostheses, lingerie, and mastectomy product accessories, including four styles of silicone gel forms. The line was created by Ruth Handler, inventor of the Barbie Doll and a breast cancer survivor herself.

Reflections
36 East 36th Street, Suite 1G
New York, NY 10016
800-300-9506 or 212-679-2160

A post-surgery boutique that accepts phone orders, accepts assignment for H.I.P. and Medicaid, and will file for Medicare reimbursements.

PROFESSIONAL ORGANIZATIONS

American College of Surgeons
633 North St. Clair Street
Chicago, IL 60611
312-202-5000
Fax: 312-202-5001
Website: www.facs.org

Will provide lists of member surgeons specializing in breast surgery in your area. Directory of Commission-Approved Cancer Programs available for a fee.

American Society of Clinical Oncology
225 Reinekers Lane, Suite #650
Alexandria, VA 22314
703-299-0150
Fax: 703-299-1040
Website: www.asco.org

A national medical specialty society representing 10,000 oncologists. The society is a leading cancer organization for scientific and educational exchange and is an active advocate on behalf of cancer patients and their healthcare providers.

American Society of Plastic and Reconstructive Surgeons
444 East Algonquin Road
Arlington Heights, IL 60005
847-228-9900 or 800-635-0635
Website: www.plasticsurgery.org

Provides written information on reconstruction, and mails a list of certified plastic and reconstructive surgeons.

Food and Drug Administration (FDA) Information Hotline
800-532-4440

Provides information regarding breast implants and answers questions about the FDA in general.

National Consortium of Breast Centers (NCBC)
P.O. Box 1334
Warsaw, IN 46581
219-267-8058

Professional membership organization of comprehensive breast centers throughout the nation.

Oncology Nursing Society
501 Holiday Drive
Pittsburgh, PA 15220-2749
412-921-7373
Fax: 412-921-6565
Website: www.ons.org

A national organization of more than 25,000 nurses dedicated to patient care, research, education, and administration in the field of oncology. Provides a variety of educational publications, audio-visual materials, and annual conferences.

Library

BOOKS AND PAMPHLETS

Advanced Breast Cancer
A Guide to Living with Metastatic Disease
Written by Musa Mayer
Edited by Linda Lamb.
O'Reilly & Associates, 1998

Few books deal specifically with metastatic cancer, or cancer that has spread beyond the breasts to other parts of the body. Musa Mayer, author of the popular book, *Examining Myself* provides a compassionate approach to the subject.

Art.Rage.Us:
Art and Writing by Women with Breast Cancer
Chronicle Books, 1998

A powerful book which demonstrates the range of emotions experienced by those affected by breast cancer. The volume includes photographs, sculpture, collages, mixed media and abstract art works along with poetry, journal entries and essays by survivors, family and others.

Ask the Doctor: Breast Cancer
Written by Vincent Freidewald, MD, and
Aman Buzdar, MD
Andrews McMeel Publishing, 1997

This book provides an easy-to-read introduction to breast cancer designed to help readers "sort through the confusing and conflicting reports that have been released to date." Recurrent icons and other design elements simplify the learning process.

Breast Cancer? Let Me Check My Schedule!
Second Edition
Edited by Peggy McCarthy and Jo An Loren
Written by Donna Cederberg, Daria Davidson, Joy Edwards, Carol Hebestreit, Betsy Lambert, Amy Langer, Cathy Masamitsu, Sally Snodgrass, Carol Stack, Carol Washington.
Foreword by Erma Bombeck.
IMEC, 1997

This dynamic book is written by ten active, professional women who share their individual experiences about what it means to live with breast cancer. All have a desire to play an active role in their treatment by being a part of the decision making process.

Breast Cancer Resource List
National Alliance of Breast Cancer Organizations (NABCO), yearly.
800-719-9154

NABCO's annual list is considered one of the best all-around guides for finding resources, including organizations and groups that can provide information, support, education, and services; help in making treatment choices; lists of publications and videos, including resources available in Spanish; information about support groups in your area; personal resources, such as places to find wigs, prostheses, and other items, and much more. An outstanding compilation of essential and hard-to-find information.

Cancer? The Facts (United Kingdom specific)
Written by Maurice Slevin and Michael Whitehouse
Oxford University Press, 1996

Includes information on diagnosis and treatment of different types of cancer, and also considers the emotional needs of cancer patients, living with advanced cancer, and the role of complementary medicine.

Cancer: A Positive Approach (U.K. specific)

Written by Hilary Thomas and Karol Sikora
Thorsons, 1995

This book aims to give information about all aspects of cancer and the treatments available so that cancer patients, their family and friends can become better informed and better able to cope with the disease. It also looks at the controversies of cancer. Includes lists of questions to ask your doctor.

Celebrating Life: African American Women Speak Out About Breast Cancer
Written by Sylvia Dunnevant
Edited by Sharon Egiebor
USFI, 1995

An intimate portrait of the breast cancer experience shared by 62 African American women. This book not only calls attention to preventive measures and treatment options, but to the affirmation of life, survival, and the human spirit.

Chemotherapy and You:
A Guide to Self Help During Treatment
National Cancer Institute, July, 1998
800-4-CANCER

A booklet, in question-and-answer format, addressing problems and concerns for patients receiving chemotherapy. Emphasis is on explanation, self-help, and participation during treatments. Includes glossary of terms and an entire section about anti-cancer drugs and drug combinations, and their side effects.

Chicken Soup for the Surviving Soul
Written by Jack Canfield, Mark Victor Hansen, Patty Aubrey, and Nancy Mitchell, R.N.
Health Communications, Inc., 1996

A special collection from the extremely popular Chicken Soup series. Stories of faith, hope and love provide inspiration and empowerment for cancer patients and their families. Outstanding contributions from Bernie Siegel, Carole King, Erma Bombeck, Norman Cousins and others.

Choices In Healing: Integrating the Best of Conventional and Complementary Approaches to Cancer
Written by Michael Lerner
MIT Press, 1994

Greeted with enthusiasm by health professionals in both the mainstream and alternative health communities, this book will be useful for those interested in considering complementary therapies in conjunction with standard medical treatment.

The Complete Guide to Homeopathy:
The Principles and Practice of Treatment
Written by Andrew Lockie, M.D. and
Nicola Geddes, M.D. with David S. Riley, M.D.
DK Publishing, 1995

An authoritative guide to this increasingly popular form of complementary medicine. The book features a photographic index of homeopathic remedies, easy-to-consult ailment charts for a wide range of common complaints, and a specially designed self-assessment questionnaire.

Confía en el Mañana: Guía para
el tratamiento del cancer de mama
Written by Vladimir Lange, MD
Lange Productions, 1999

The Spanish language version of Be a Survivor.™ This book is not simply a translation; it has been rewritten to reflect the attitudes and needs of Latina women and their families, and features excerpts from Latina breast cancer survivors.

Dr. Susan Love's Breast Book
Second Edition
Written by Susan M. Love, M.D. with Karen Lindsey
Addison-Wesley Publishing, 1995

A well-known and respected breast surgeon and feminist discusses all conditions of the breast, from benign to malignant. Complete general reference on all breast health topics.

Eating Hints: Tips and Recipes for Better
Nutrition During Cancer Treatment
National Cancer Institute, June, 1997.
800-4-CANCER

The National Cancer Institute (NCI) has prepared this booklet to help you learn more about your diet needs and eating problems.

Examining Myself
Written by Musa Mayer
Faber & Faber, 1994

A beautifully crafted, deeply personal account of one woman's experience with breast cancer. The writer weaves in useful medical information, making this a book well worth reading.

Facing Forward:
A Guide for Cancer Survivors
National Cancer Institute, February, 1996
800-4-CANCER

Addresses the special needs of cancer survivors and their families, focusing on four major areas of need: maintaining physical health, addressing emotional concerns, managing insurance issues, and handling employment problems. Resource numbers are given for each category.

For Single Women With Breast Cancer
Y-ME National Breast Organization, 1995
800-221-2141

Many women contributed to the writing of this booklet, which strives to offer practical guidance and emotional support to single women facing breast cancer therapy, and to convey the message that they are not alone.

Living Beyond Limits
Written by David Spiegel, M.D.
A Fawcett Columbine Book,
Published by Ballantine Books, 1994

Based on fifteen years of groundbreaking research,
Dr. Spiegel outlines a scientifically-proven program to
help all people with chronic illnesses enhance the quality
of their lives. Recognizing the essential healing connection between body and mind, he teaches how to:

• Face the shattering diagnosis head-on
• Deal directly with fears of dying
• Build and sustain networks of support
• Review and reorder life's priorities
• Strengthen family relationships
• Improve communications with doctors
• Master pain through self-hypnosis

An outstanding and inspiring book.

Love, Medicine and Miracles
Written by Bernie Siegel, M.D.
Perennial Library, 1990

Promotes visualization, meditation, discussion, and
peace of mind. Emphasizes the healing power of
unconditional love and the influence patients can have
over their own recovery. A landmark book by a surgeon and renowned thought-leader on the subject of
patient empowerment and mind/body unity. Also
available in CD-ROM format.

No Less A Woman:
Femininity, Sexuality & Breast Cancer
Written by Deborah Hobble Kahane, M.S.W.
Hunter House Publishing, 1995

A positive look at breast cancer that helps those diagnosed feel less alone in their feelings and their fears. It
is a valuable tool that helps women get through the
breast cancer experience by hearing from those who
have already been there.

Sexuality & Cancer: For the Woman
Who Has Cancer, and Her Partner
Written by Leslie R. Schover, Ph.D.
American Cancer Society, 1996
800-ACS-2345

This booklet contains information about cancer and
sexuality in the areas that most concern you and your
partner. The information provided is devised to allow
you and your partner to openly discuss your sex life
together.

Sharing: A Family's Guide To Breast Cancer
Bristol-Myers Squibb Co., 1994

Discusses the emotional side of coping with breast cancer. It is intended to help family members better
understand their own reactions and their loved ones'
response to a diagnosis of breast cancer. Eloquently
written and beautifully laid out. Available through your
oncologist's office or your physician's Bristol-Myers
Squibb representative.

Sharing: A Woman's Guide To Breast Cancer
Bristol-Myers Squibb Co., 1994

This booklet is intended to help women share their
feelings about a breast cancer diagnosis with the people
who are close the them. One of the best publications
on this topic. Available through your oncologist's office
or your physician's Bristol-Myers Squibb representative.

*Taking Time: Support for People With Cancer
and the People Who Care About Them*
National Cancer Institute, 1990
800-4-CANCER

This book is written as a guide for the patient and her
loved ones to help them cope with their fears and deal
with their feelings upon being diagnosed with cancer. It
teaches everyone concerned to define their feelings about
cancer by creating a positive and loving environment in
which to continue living as normally as possible.

What You Need to Know About Breast Cancer
National Cancer Institute, 1998
800-4-CANCER

NCI's comprehensive pamphlet on breast cancer covers
symptoms, diagnosis, treatment, emotional issues, and
questions to ask your doctor. Includes a glossary of
terms.

When the Woman You Love Has Breast Cancer
Written by Larry Eiler
Queen Bee Publishing, 1994

Based on the personal experiences of the author, this
book addresses issues faced by a man whose wife and
friend has breast cancer, and the steps he can take to be
supportive.

When The Woman You Love Has Breast Cancer
Y-ME National Breast Cancer Organization, 1997
800-221-2141

Y-ME has created this booklet to help partners provide
emotional support to their loved ones. Single copies are
available at no charge.

*A Woman's Decision:
Breast Care, Treatment, & Reconstruction
Second Edition*
Written by Karen Berger and John Bostwick III, M.D.
Quality Medical Publishing, 1994

A sensitive and authoritative book that will help women
assess their options, familiarize themselves with the
techniques used in treating cancer, and prepare themselves for what to expect medically and emotionally
from reconstructive surgery. Copiously illustrated with
outstanding photographs and drawings.

*A Woman's Guide to Breast Cancer
Diagnosis and Treatment*
California Dept. of Health Services,
Breast Cancer Early Detection Program, 1995
Available from: Breast Cancer Treatment Options,
Medical Board of California
1426 Howe Ave., Suite 54
Sacramento, CA 95825

This booklet is an invaluable guide for the woman who
has been diagnosed with breast cancer. A comprehensive overview of all the stages a woman is likely to
encounter as she goes from diagnosis to treatment and
recovery. Elegant illustrations complement the clearly
written and beautifully laid out text. Sidebars summa-
rize information, call out important concepts, and list
commonly asked questions.

California law mandates that this publication be given
to the patient at the time of biopsy, but every woman
facing breast cancer should obtain a copy.

VIDEOS AND CD-ROMS

*Assessing Your Risk for Breast Cancer:
There is Something You Can Do*
Video - 20 minutes
Zeneca Pharmaceuticals, 1999

This video discusses risk factors for breast cancer and helps women identify if they may benefit from prophylactic treatment with Tamoxifen. A diverse group of survivors are represented and the video comes complete with an educational brochure and a card to fill out and take to your doctor.

*Be a Survivor™: An Overview
of Breast Cancer Treatment*
Video - 28 minutes
Lange Productions, 1999
888-LANGE-88

The video companion to the *Be a Survivor™*
CD-ROM and to this book.

The program, clearly illustrated with 3-D animated graphics, gives a step-by-step presentation of the treatment process, from needle biopsy to nipple reconstruction. Highlighted with comments from breast cancer survivors, this video is an ideal take-home guide for newly-diagnosed patients.

*Be a Survivor™: Your Interactive Guide
to Breast Cancer Treatment*
CD-ROM
Lange Productions, 1999
888-LANGE-88

This multi-award winning CD-ROM is the program on which this book is based. It allows you to actually see the procedures and the 3-D animated graphics, and to hear the patient interviews. You can explore the CD-ROM at your own pace, and print out lists of resources or questions to ask your healthcare professionals.

The program features more than twelve hours of material, including sections on both standard and complementary therapies, breast anatomy, diagnosis and staging, breast cancer resources, help for the patient's life partner, and life after cancer.

The CD-ROM, designed for users who are not computer experts, is extremely easy to use: any topic can be accessed with a simple click of the mouse. On some computers, you can use the program by simply touching the screen with your finger.

Breast Facts, The Basics
Video - 8 minutes
Lange Productions, 1998
888-LANGE-88

This videotape provides an excellent introduction to breast health by describing breast anatomy and physiology, breast lumps, "fibrocystic disease," and factors that may contribute to the risk of breast cancer.

Breast Reconstruction
Video - 17 minutes
Mentor H/S, Inc., 1999
800-525-0245

This patient education video is designed to facilitate patient understanding of breast augmentation and breast reconstruction. The video discusses the various options available in these procedures, types of breast implants, the actual surgery, benefits, potential risks, and complications.

B.S.E For Teens — with Jennie Garth Introduction
Video - 7 minutes
Lange Productions, 1997
888-LANGE-88

This program encourages teenagers to learn how breasts look and feel now, when they are healthy, so that they will be more likely to spot a change later on.

Beautiful 3-D graphics illustrate breast anatomy, while an all-teen, multi-ethnic cast clearly demonstrate the latest techniques for breast self examination. Upbeat tempo, unconventional editing, and an introduction by actress Jennie Garth of Beverly Hills 90210, make this video a hit with teenage audiences.

A valuable teaching tool for daughters of women who have been diagnosed with breast cancer.

Companion Video to the Be a Survivor Book
Video - 35 minutes
Lange Productions, 1999
888-LANGE-88

Women who have "been there" share their stories. The perfect companion to the Be a Survivor book, this video brings to life the survivors you've read here with on-screen interviews about their triumphs over breast cancer.

Confia en el Mañana
Video - 40 minutes
Lange Productions, 1999
888-LANGE-88

This video is based on the Be a Survivor™ video, but is not simply a translation. The program has been completely rewritten to reflect the attitudes and needs of Latina women and their families. Features all Latina survivors.

Love, Medicine and Miracles
by Bernie Siegel, M.D.
CD-ROM
HarperCollins Publishers, 1997

The CD-ROM version of Dr. Siegel's highly successful book promotes visualization, meditation, discussion, and peace of mind. Outstanding informative and entertaining tool that can be enjoyed on many levels.

Includes features on picture therapy, laughter therapy, a personal workbook, and much more. It's like a personal workshop or house call by Dr. Siegel.

The New B.S.E. with Marriette Hartley
Video - 6 minutes
Lange Productions, 1999
888-LANGE-88

This much-acclaimed video follows the latest American Cancer Society guidelines. Easy to follow demonstrations use 3-D graphics and feature women of a variety of ages and ethnic backgrounds. The program stresses the importance of monthly B.S.E. as part of a breast health routine, and encourages patients to adopt this lifesaving habit.

A must for all women, and particularly for close relatives of women diagnosed with breast cancer. Also available in Spanish, Korean, Russian, Ukranian, and Slovak.

Quality Mammography Can Save Your Life
Video - 8 minutes
Lange Productions, 1997
888-LANGE-88

This "must see" video emphasizes that mammography, in combination with breast self examination and clinical examination, can lead to early detection and improve chances of successful treatment. The program outlines the most current recommendations on frequency of mammography — every year for all women, starting at age forty, or starting ten years younger than the age at which a close relative was diagnosed with breast cancer.

Glossary

abscess
A pocket of pus caused by an infection.

AC
Chemotherapy combination of two different drugs: Adriamycin and Cytoxan.

Adriamycin (doxorubicin)
A drug used to kill cancer cells.

Adrucil (5-fluorouracil)
A drug used to kill cancer cells.

anesthesia
Procedure used to make surgery painless, either by local numbing or by putting the patient to sleep. It is usually performed by an anesthesiologist or a nurse anesthetist.

antiemetic
A medicine that relieves nausea (feeling sick to the stomach) and vomiting (throwing up).

antihistamine
Medication used to relieve the symptoms of allergies.

antioxidant
Compounds which slow the deterioration (or oxidation) of cells in the body. Vitamins C and E, as well as beta-carotene are antioxidants.

Arimidex (anastrozole)
A drug for treatment of advanced breast cancer in postmenopausal women (women who have stopped having their periods).

aspiration
Removal of liquid or tissue cells from a cyst or other structure in the breast, by inserting a needle and drawing (aspirating) fluid into a syringe.

bank blood
Blood that has been donated and stored for later use.

beta-carotene
An antioxidant which is stored and converted into Vitamin A by the body.

bilateral
Something that is present on both sides of the body. For example, a bilateral mastectomy is a surgery where both breasts are removed.

blood cell count
A test that measures the number of red blood cells (RBC's), white blood cells (WBC's), and platelets in a blood sample. In addition to providing other information, this test helps evaluate the effect of chemotherapy on the bone marrow where the blood cells are produced.

blood transfusion
The transfer of blood into a patient during surgery.

bone marrow transplant
A procedure in which bone marrow is extracted and then transplanted back into the body after large doses of chemotherapy have been given.

brachytherapy
A form of radiation therapy in which the source of the radiation is placed close to, or implanted in, the body.

breast form
Something with the shape and texture of a breast, created with tissue or with a prosthetic.

CAF
Chemotherapy combination of three different drugs: Cytoxan, Adriamycin, and 5-fluorouracil.

carbohydrate
A chemical compound which serves as a basic source of energy. Foods high in carbohydrates include sugars and starches such as bread and pasta.

carcinoembryonic antigen (CEA)
Blood test used to follow women with metastatic breast cancer to help determine if the treatments are working.

carcinogen
Any substance that initiates or promotes the development of cancer.

carcinoma
a form of cancer that develops in the lining of the organs of the body, such as the skin, the uterus, the lungs, or the breast.

carcinoma in situ
A carcinoma still in an early stage of development when the cancer has not spread outside the area where it began.

catheter
A tube used to allow fluid to pass into or out of the body.

cell
The basic building block of all organisms. Individual cells can only be seen when they are magnified through a microscope.

CFP
Chemotherapy combination of three different drugs: Cytoxan, 5-fluorouracil, and prednisone.

chromosome
One of the many strands of DNA material within the cell that carries genetic information.

circulatory system
The system consisting of the heart and blood vessels which provides blood to all parts of the body.

CMF
Chemotherapy combination of three different drugs: Cytoxan, methotrexate, and 5-fluorouracil.

CMFVP
Chemotherapy combination of five different drugs: Cytoxan, methotrexate, 5-fluorouracil, Vincristine, and prednisone.

colony stimulating factors
Chemotherapy additives which stimulate the bone marrow. May be required to maintain adequate blood cell counts during chemotherapy treatment.

combination chemotherapy
Use of two or more chemicals to achieve maximum damage to tumor cells. Most common include: *CAF, CFP, CMF,* and *CMFVP*

cyclophosphamide (Cytoxan or Neosar)
A drug used to kill cancer cells.

cyst
A sac-like structure that contains liquid or semi-solid material.

Cytoxan (cyclophosphamide)
A drug used to kill cancer cells.

DCIS
Abbreviation for ductal carcinoma *in situ.*

dietitian
A credentialed professional specializing in diets and nutrition.

DNA
Material found in the nucleus of all cells. Contains genetic information for cell division and cell growth.

donor site
That part of the body from which tissue is taken for transfer to another part of the body for reconstruction.

double blind
A research study in which neither the participants nor the researchers know which subjects are in the control group and which subjects are in the test group.

doubling time
The time required to double the number of cells in a group of cells or in a tumor. A short doubling time (under 100 days) indicates a fast-growing tumor.

doxorubicin (Adriamycin)
A drug used to kill cancer cells.

drain
A plastic tube, usually attached to a bulb, placed into the surgical site to collect any draining blood or fluid for a few days following surgery.

ductal carcinoma in situ
A cancer inside breast ducts that has not grown through the wall of the duct into the surrounding tissues. Also known simply as DCIS.

early detection
Taking the necessary steps to discovering cancer as early as possible, including monthly breast self-examination, yearly clinical breast examination by a healthcare provider, and mammography.

edema
Excess fluid in a body part. Usually makes it appear swollen or puffy. Lymphedema is swelling of the arm as a result of scarring of the lymph ducts after radiation or surgery in the axilla.

electron beam
The stream of energy used to administer radiation therapy.

estrogen
A female hormone secreted by the ovaries which is essential for menstruation, reproduction, and the development of secondary sex characteristics, such as breasts.

FAC
Chemotherapy combination of three different drugs: 5-fluorouracil, Adriamycin, and Cytoxan.

fibroadenoma
A noncancerous, solid tumor most commonly found in breasts of younger women.

fibroid
A tumor composed of fibers or fibrous tissues.

5-FU (5-fluorouracil)
A drug used to kill cancer cells.

flap
A portion of tissue with its blood supply moved from one part of the body to another. Flaps of muscle, fat, and skin are frequently used to provide tissue for reconstructing breasts.

general anesthesia
Anesthesia which puts your whole body to sleep. Usually given through injection or by breathing in gases.

genes
Areas on chromosomes that contain hereditary information that is transferred from cell to cell.

guided imagery
Using directed mental images to provide relaxation, mental healing, or higher levels of consciousness.

hemoglobin
A protein in blood which carries oxygen.

HER-2/neu
An oncogene which may help determine resistance to hormone and chemotherapy.

hereditary
Passed from generation to generation in a family.

hormone
Chemical substance that helps regulate growth, metabolism, and reproduction.

immune system
System by which the body protects itself from outside invaders or internal defects.

infiltrating ductal carcinoma
A cancer that began in a milk duct and has spread to areas outside the duct.

lactation
Milk production in the breasts.

LCIS
Abbreviation for lobular carcinoma in situ.

lesion
A diseased area of tissue.

linear accelerator
A machine that produces high energy x-ray beams to destroy cancer cells during radiation therapy.

lobular carcinoma in situ
A tumor confined to the milk-producing lobules of the breast (LCIS).

margin
The area of normal tissue surrounding a tumor when it is surgically removed.

metastatic cancer
Cancer which has spread beyond the breast to other parts of the body.

methotrexate
A drug used to kill cancer cells.

micro-surgery
Sewing together almost hair-thin blood vessels with the aid of a microscope.

mind-body connection
A philosophical theory that states that the mind can control bodily functions.

modified radical mastectomy
The most common type of mastectomy. Breast skin, nipple, areola, and some of the underarm lymph nodes are removed. The chest muscles are saved.

myo-cutaneous flap
A section of muscle, fat, and skin transferred for reconstruction of the breast.

needle localization
A procedure in which a radiologist pinpoints a tumor with a special mammography unit, then inserts a thin wire into the breast. Later, a surgeon will follow this wire to find the tumor.

neurotransmitter
A chemical agent that can act as a natural mood enhancer or pain reliever in the body.

Nolvadex (tamoxifen)
An anti-estrogen drug that may be given to women with estrogen receptor positive tumors, to slow or stop tumor growth.

non-surgical biopsy
A biopsy where samples of a lump or tumor are removed with a needle under local anesthesia.

norepinephrine
A neurotransmitter which has adrenaline-like affects on the body.

oncogene
A gene that contributes to the malignant transformation of a cell.

oncologist
A physician who specializes in cancer treatment.

oncology
Medical specialty dealing with cancer treatment.

osteoporosis
Increased bone fragility that occurs with age, often due to lack of the female hormone estrogen.

paclitaxel (Taxol)
A drug used to kill cancer cells.

PDQ
A source of information published by the National Cancer Institute which lists all clinical and experimental trials currently underway.

pectoralis muscles
Muscles located under the breast and attached to the front of the chest wall and extending to the upper arms.

PICC line
A vascular access device inserted through the skin of the forearm, so that chemotherapy can be injected without danger of leakage under the skin, or damage to the vein.

ploidy
The number of chromosome sets in a cell.

port
A vascular access device surgically inserted under the skin of the chest, and connected to a very large vein, so that chemotherapy can be injected without damage to the veins.

precancerous lesions
Abnormal cellular changes that are potentially capable of becoming cancer.

prednisone - (Deltasone, Meticorten, Orasone)
A steroid used to decrease inflammation; also used in combination with cytotoxic drugs.

progesterone
A female hormone produced by the ovaries during a specific time in the menstrual cycle that causes the uterus to prepare for pregnancy and the breasts to prepare to produce milk.

prognosis
A prediction of the course of the disease; the future prospect for the patient.

prosthesis
An artificial breast form worn inside a bra after a mastectomy.

protein
Complex compounds which hold amino acids essential for growth and repair of tissues. High protein foods include meat, fish, nuts, and legumes.

radical mastectomy
Removal of entire breast, as well as underlying muscles, causing significant deformity. No longer performed today.

recurrence
Reappearance of cancer after a period of remission.

risk counselor
A trained healthcare professional who can advise a woman on her risk of developing breast cancer.

saline
A salt water solution,
1. given intravenously during surgery to maintain proper body functioning, or
2. used to fill a synthetic implant for breast reconstruction.

second opinion
A diagnosis given by another doctor.

sentinel node
The single axillary lymph node that can be examined to determine if cancer has spread beyond the breast to other lymph nodes.

serotonin
A neurotransmitter that has a calming, pain killing effect on the body.

stem cell
Cells which will eventually become blood cell producers in the bone marrow.

stem cell rescue
Same as bone marrow transplant.

stereotactic core needle biopsy
A biopsy performed using two mammographic views to pinpoint the site of the tumor.

stereotactic unit
Special mammography equipment which enables a radiologist to place a biopsy needle precisely into a tumor.

suppressor gene
A gene that can reverse the effect of a specific type of mutation in other genes.

suture
A surgeon's stitch.

tamoxifen (Nolvadex)
An anti-estrogen drug that may be given to women with estrogen receptor positive tumors to block tumor cell growth.

Taxol (paclitaxel)
A drug used for treatment of breast cancer

toxins
Chemicals from food and the environment that collect in the body and diminish its ability to function properly.

"tummy tuck"
A procedure in which a portion of fat and skin is removed from the abdomen, reducing the size of one's "tummy." It is performed as part of the TRAM flap reconstruction procedure.

ultrasound
High frequency sound waves used to locate a tumor inside the body. Helps determine if a breast lump is solid or filled with fluid.

ultrasound-guided biopsy
The use of ultrasound to guide a biopsy needle to obtain a sample of tissue for analysis by a pathologist.

visualization
Forming a mental image of something not present to the sight. This technique can be used for relaxation or to help your body fight cancer.

Zoladex (goserelin acetate implant)
A drug for treatment of advanced breast cancer in premenopausal and perimenopausal women.

QUESTIONS TO ASK YOUR HEALTHCARE PROVIDERS

The following are questions gathered from throughout the book. They are broken down by chapter with space for you to write down your answers and make your own notes. Feel free to tear or cut out these pages for the person who will be accompanying you on your medical visits.

CHAPTER 1: FACING BREAST CANCER

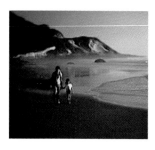

Questions to Ask Your Doctor:

What should I tell my loved ones about my condition?

May I bring members of my family, or a friend, to talk to you directly?

Can you refer me to a counselor or to a support group specializing in breast cancer issues?

Can you give me the name of a breast cancer expert who can give me a second opinion?

Could you forward my chart, test results, and my biopsy slides to the doctor who is going to give me a second opinion?

Could you give me the names of specialists you think I should see??

How about another set of names so I can choose the specialist(s) I like best?

Is there a multidisciplinary breast cancer team in the facility where you practice?

Tell me about your, or your colleagues' experience in dealing with breast cancer.

*Do you have any pamphlets, videos, or CD-ROMs about breast cancer that
we can take home and review?*

Do you, or your clinic or hospital, have a resource center? A library?

Can you refer me to breast cancer groups or organizations in this area?

Where can I find more information about breast cancer?

Your Notes:

Chapter 4: Surgery - lumpectomy

Questions to Ask Your Anesthesiologist:

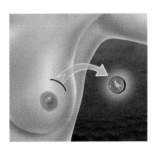

If I have general anesthesia, how long will it take me to get back to normal?

What will I feel and hear if I have local anesthesia?

*Will you give me something to control the pain after I wake up from
the anesthetic?*

Questions to Ask Your Surgeon:

Is lumpectomy an option for me? Why or why not?

How much breast tissue will be removed?

How will my breast look after the treatment? Can you show me pictures?

Where, and how big will the scar be?

How much pain should I expect in the first few days after the procedure?

Do I need to arrange to have someone come help me with daily activities?

How long before I can go back to my regular work or leisure activities?

Will there be any long term effects?

Your Notes:

CHAPTER 4: SURGERY - MASTECTOMY

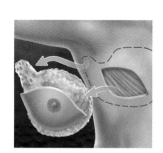

Questions to Ask Your Anesthesiologist:

Will you give me something to help me relax before surgery?

How long will it take me to get back to normal after a general anesthetic?

What are the side effects of anesthesia?

Questions to Ask Your Surgeon:

Is lumpectomy an option for me? Why or why not?

Does a mastectomy decrease the chances of the cancer coming back?

How much pain should I expect in the first few days after the procedure?

What can I do to relieve the pain?

Do I need to arrange to have someone help me with my daily activities?

How long before I can go back to my regular work or leisure activities?

How will I look after a mastectomy if I decide against reconstruction?

Can you show me pictures?

Can you refer me to a plastic surgeon so I can discuss my reconstruction options?

What kind of reconstruction procedure do you think would be best for me?

Who can I talk to about my concerns about appearance, dating, pregnancy, etc?

CHAPTER 5: RECONSTRUCTION

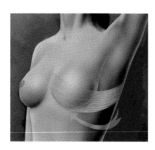

Questions to Ask Your Plastic Surgeon:

What type of reconstruction do you think is best for me?

Will an implant make it more difficult to detect a local recurrence?

Can you show me pictures of reconstruction procedures you have done?

Could I meet with some of the women so I can see and feel their breasts?

Will my insurance pay for the reconstruction, even if it is done later?

Will I have a lot of pain? How can the pain be treated?

Questions to Ask Your Insurance Company:

Does my policy cover the costs of the implant surgery, the implant anesthesia, and other related hospital costs? To what extent?

Does it cover treatments for medical problems that may be caused by the implant or the reconstruction?

Does it cover removal of the implants if this becomes necessary?

If I choose to delay reconstruction and my company changes insurance plans, will I still be covered for breast reconstruction at a later date?

Chapter 6: Radiation Therapy

Questions to Ask Your Doctor:

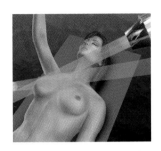

Why do I need radiation therapy?

How is the radiation oncologist (physician) involved if the treatments are given by the therapists?

How will I evaluate the effectiveness of the treatments?

Can I continue my usual work or exercise schedule?

Can I miss a few treatments?

Can I arrange to be treated elsewhere if I am traveling?

What side effects, if they occur, should I report immediately?

Can I expose the treated area to the sun?

Will I be able to conceive and bear a child after treatments?

Your Notes:

CHAPTER 7: CHEMOTHERAPY

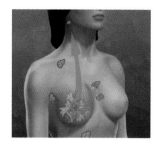

Questions to Ask Your Doctor:

Do I need chemotherapy? Why?

What drugs do you recommend?

What are the benefits and risks of chemotherapy?

How successful is this treatment for the type of cancer I have?

How will you evaluate the effectiveness of the treatments?

What side effects will I experience?

Can I work while I'm having chemotherapy?

Can I travel between treatments (short business or pleasure trips)?

What other limitations can I expect?

How can I manage nausea?

Will I be given medications to treat side effects?

Can I take public transportation home after treatments?

Should I eat before I come for my treatments?

Can I take vitamins or herbs if I choose?

Will I continue to have my menstrual periods? If not, when will they return?

Should I use birth control? What type do you recommend?

Will I be able to conceive and bear a child after treatments?

Your Notes:

CHAPTER 8: HORMONAL THERAPY

Questions to Ask your Doctor:

Did the tests on my tumor show that the cells were sensitive to hormones? (Estrogen Receptor Positive, or Progesterone Receptor Positive)

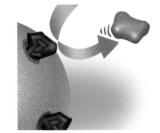

Should I be treated with hormonal therapy or with chemotherapy, and why?

How will it affect my chance to have children?

How will it affect my sexual function?

What side effects should I expect?

Can I get pregnant while taking tamoxifen?

What birth control method would be most suitable to my lifestyle?

What is the latest research data on the safety of tamoxifen?

What is the latest research data on how long to take tamoxifen?

Your Notes:

CHAPTER 10: CLINICAL TRIALS

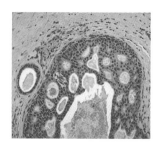

Questions to Ask About a Clinical Trial:

What is involved in terms of tests, treatments, and additional time commitments?

What results can be reasonably expected in my particular case?

What are the currently accepted treatments and how do they compare to the trial?

What would my financial commitment be and how can I cope with it?

Will I need to be available for follow-up testing indefinitely?

CHAPTER 11: LIFE AFTER CANCER

Questions to Ask Your Doctor or Nurse:

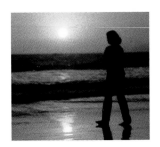

What can I do if I wake up at night worrying about my cancer?

Will the cancer cells that may have spread to other parts of my body start to grow when I stop taking chemotherapy?

What can I do about feeling excessively tired?

Why have I lost interest in intimate relations with my partner?

Why can't I sleep or relax or feel interested in anything?

Why can't I stop feeling that I am going to die because of the cancer?

Your Notes:

CHAPTER 12: A GUIDE FOR YOUR PARTNER

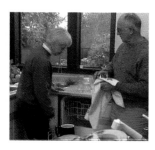

Questions to Ask Her Doctor:

Do you have any pamphlets, videos, or CD-ROMs about breast cancer that we can take home and review?

Is there a Resource Center or patient library in the facility where you practice?

Who would you recommend we see for a second opinion?

Can you put us in touch with women who you treated for breast cancer, and with their partners?

Will there be loss of sensation in the breast area?

Will chemotherapy cause her hair to fall out?

Can we see pictures of what the surgical scar could look like?

Index

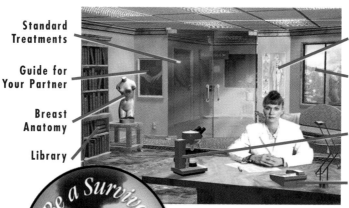
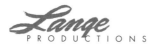

Be a Survivor™
THE COMPLETE PROGRAM

Three ways
to reinforce information

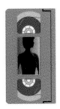

SEE THE VIDEO... A crystal-clear overview of everything you need to know on day one. Watch it in the healthcare provider's office or take it home to view with your family.

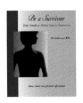

READ THE BOOK... A readily-accessible source of "must have" information, including questions to ask your healthcare providers.

EXPLORE THE CD ROM... Detailed description of all phases of therapy, from biopsy to nipple reconstruction, to be used throughout treatment and recovery. Just point and click!

Additional Resources available from Lange Productions:
The New BSE with Mariette Hartley
BSE for Teens with Jenny Garth
Quality Mammography Can Save Your Life
Un Toque Saludable-Early Detection for Latina Women

NO NEWLY-DIAGNOSED WOMAN
SHOULD GO HOME EMPTY-HANDED !

ASK YOUR HEALTHCARE PROVIDER
ABOUT THESE PROGRAMS OR CALL
1-888-LANGE-88

Be a Survivor™ Book, Video and CD-ROM

"This book does for the breast cancer survivor's mind what Chicken Soup does for the survivor's soul."

JACK CANFIELD, *Author*
Chicken Soup for the Surviving Soul

"Women and their partners will get a lot out of this CD-ROM. [It has] 12 hours of fact-packed information, given in scientific and lay terms."

JOURNAL OF THE
NATIONAL CANCER INSTITUTE

"Lives up to its title, and more. Geared toward breast cancer patients, their families and their support people, this CD-ROM could make all the difference in the attitude, and thus the recovery, of the patient facing breast cancer."

ADVANCE: FOR RADIOLOGIC
SCIENCE PROFESSIONALS

"A long-overdue book... 'One-stop shopping' for up-to-date, objective information that women need to make confident, informed decisions."

BETSY MULLEN, *survivor*
Founder, President, and CEO
WIN Against Breast Cancer

"A useful tool for patients and any lay person interested in breast cancer."

JOURNAL OF THE
AMERICAN MEDICAL ASSOCIATION

"An authoritative guide, illustrated with candid thoughts of breast cancer survivors."

WILLIAM H. GOODSON III, M.D.
Breast Surgeon

"A positive presentation of the essential facts every patient needs to know. Equally useful for the nurse and the family."

AMERICAN JOURNAL OF NURSING

"An excellent program that should help women face the difficult issues of cancer."

AMAN U. BUZDAR, M.D., *Author*
Ask the Doctor: Breast Cancer
M.D. Anderson Cancer Center

"The latest in the fight against breast cancer is as close as your home computer, and could save your life. It's realistic. It's informative. It's powerful. It's all on the new CD-ROM called "Be A Survivor.""

FOX NEWS

"For those ready to launch an all-out attack, Be A Survivor is a most empowering roadmap through the medical forest. It demystifies this disease. ...A loving guidebook through uncharted waters."

DOTTY EWING
Member of the Board,
WIN Against Breast Cancer